SUPPLE BODY

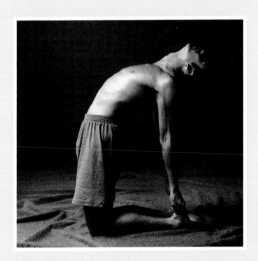

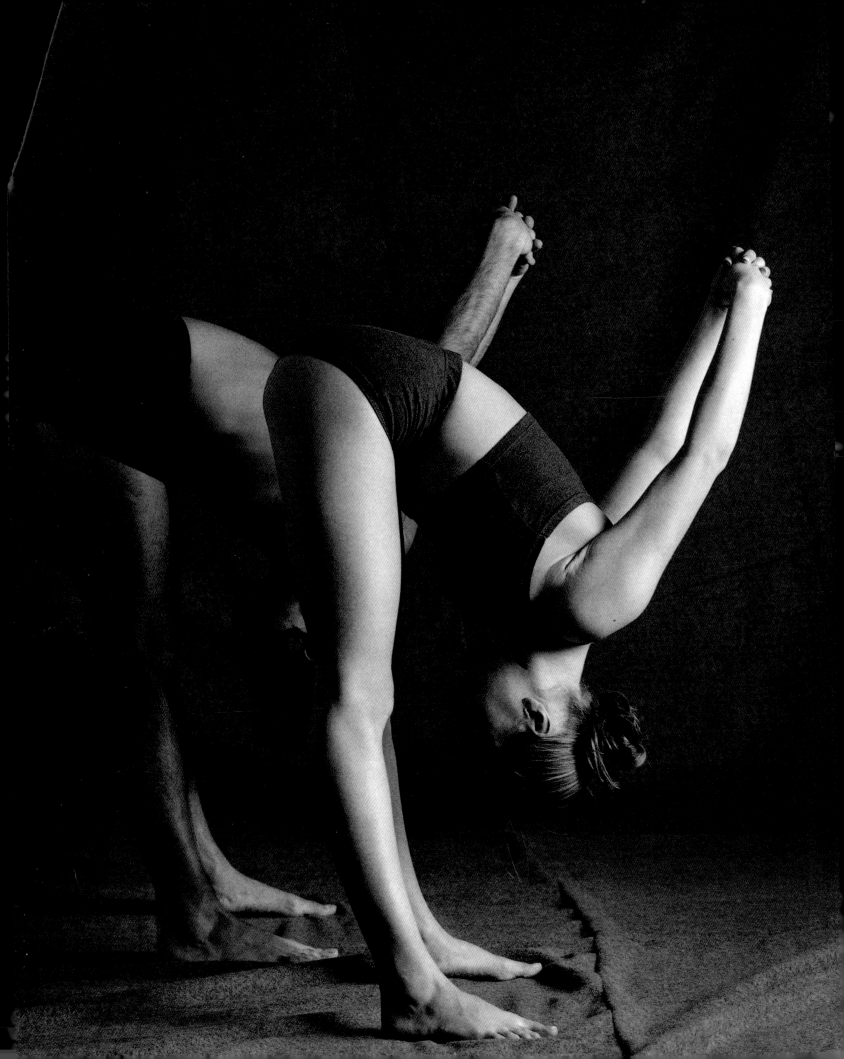

SUPPLE BODY

The new way to fitness, strength and flexibility

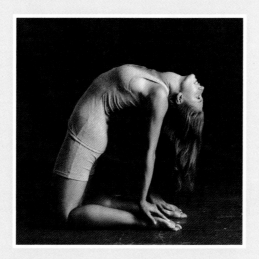

Sara Black

Photography by Antonia Deutsch

DUNCAN BAIRD PUBLISHERS

LONDON

The Supple Body

This edition first published in 1999 by
Duncan Baird Publishers
Sixth Floor
Castle House
75–76 Wells Street
London
W1P 3RE

A CIP catalogue listing for this book is
available from the British Library

ISBN 1-900131-22-6

Designer: Sue Bush
Consultant physiotherapists: Sarah Clark,
Liliana Djurovic (see page 144)
Consultant editor: Stephanie Schwartz
Editors: Peter Bently, Judy Dean
Commissioned photography: Antonia Deutsch
Commissioned artwork: Ron Hayward
Models: Ruth Warrior, Paul Baldwin
Studio adviser: Ian Driver
Indexers: Tom Loxley, Clare Richards

Cover design: Sonya Merali
Photographs: Antonia Deutsch

Typeset in Metaplus
Colour reproduction by Bright Arts, Hong Kong
Photographic prints by Metro Imaging Ltd
Printed in Singapore

10 9 8 7 6 5 4 3 2 1

Contents

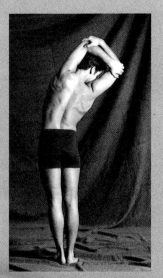

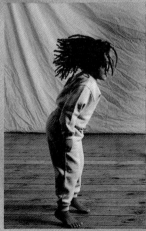

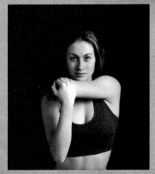

Introduction

Over a short period it is easy to free yourself from stresses and tensions and begin to unlock your body. When your body is supple and relaxed, you will feel better physically and mentally, with a clearer and more focused mind and a lighter spirit. This requires a new approach to exercise that combines the best contemporary thinking on fitness and flexibility with the essence of many non-Western philosophies.

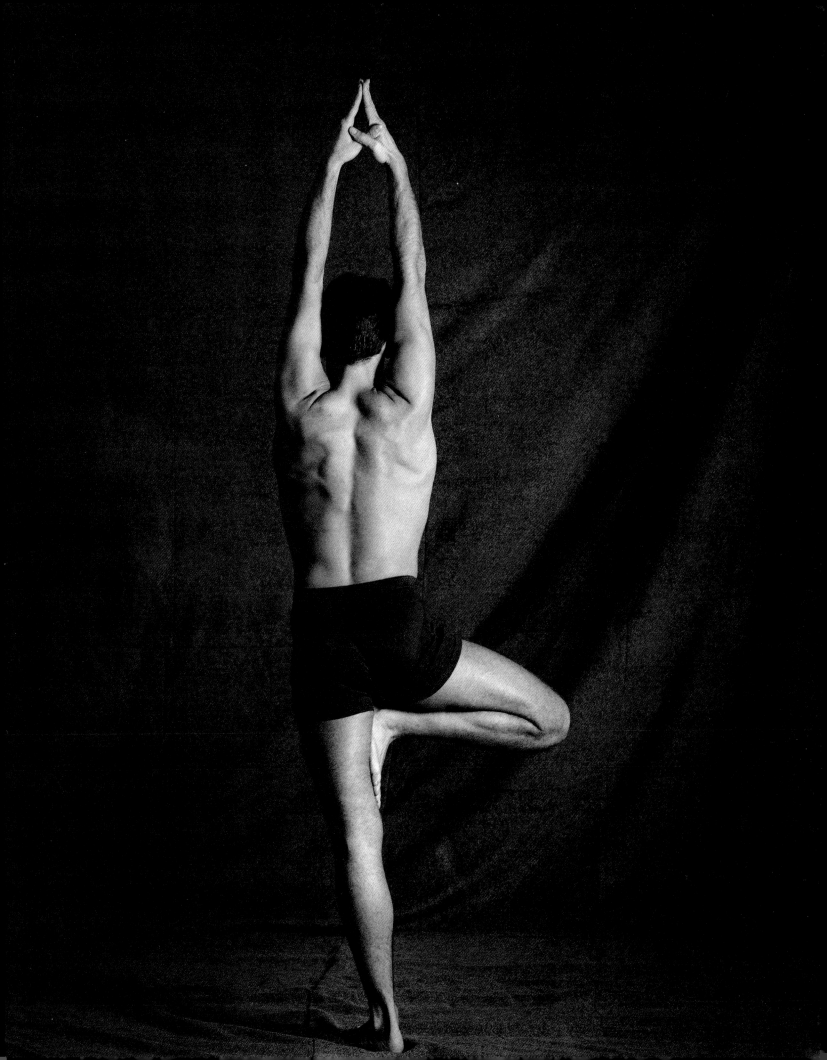

The philosophy of fitness

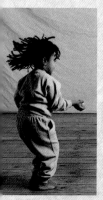
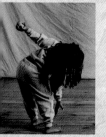
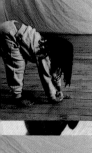
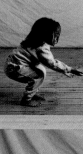
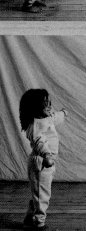

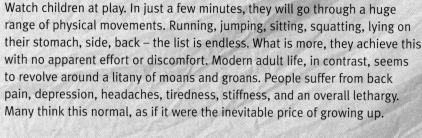
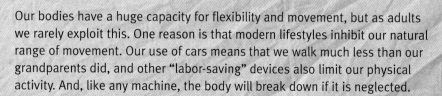

Remember when you were a kid. You had boundless energy and a body that you took for granted. You would run all day, jump over fences, climb trees, and generally do all the things that children do without a thought about your body. You would never have believed then that one day your body could be stiff or that your stamina might not last.

Watch children at play. In just a few minutes, they will go through a huge range of physical movements. Running, jumping, sitting, squatting, lying on their stomach, side, back – the list is endless. What is more, they achieve this with no apparent effort or discomfort. Modern adult life, in contrast, seems to revolve around a litany of moans and groans. People suffer from back pain, depression, headaches, tiredness, stiffness, and an overall lethargy. Many think this normal, as if it were the inevitable price of growing up.

Physical movement is still central to the way most of us live our lives. You probably have no idea how many times you get up from a chair each day, because it is something that happens so often. Yet this simple act uses over 200 different muscles and is a miracle of balance and coordination. Why is it then that so many of us, somewhere between our childhood and the present day, have lost the effortless grace and energy that we once had?

Our bodies have a huge capacity for flexibility and movement, but as adults we rarely exploit this. One reason is that modern lifestyles inhibit our natural range of movement. Our use of cars means that we walk much less than our grandparents did, and other "labor-saving" devices also limit our physical activity. And, like any machine, the body will break down if it is neglected.

As we go through life, we acquire tension in the body through physical and emotional pain. Injuries as ordinary as a twisted ankle or as dramatic as a slipped disk leave their marks even after they have been cured; and the emotional trials of our daily lives show up in raised shoulders and defensively-hunched backs. Often we accept this tension as normal and forget that we ever had a capacity for movement without it. With a little time and concentrated effort, it is easy to change this state of affairs and to benefit from the body's full and natural potential. The Olympic athlete has a child's flexibility and an adult's mental and physical strength – a perfect example of someone who has harnessed and maximized the body's potential. To realize possibilities that have been dormant for too long, you must look within yourself. Learning to understand how your body works can unlock its potential to improve your fitness. This book will help you to do just that.

the Eastern aspects of modern exercise

So many people believe that the body must suffer in order to become fitter because, in the West, mind and body have been separated. The age-old tradition of brain versus brawn dictates that if you use your mind, then the body is weak; on the other hand, if your body is strong, the mind is weak. But to achieve a balanced healthy lifestyle, the two cannot be separated.

This confusion does not exist in many Eastern disciplines. The idea that a healthy body requires a healthy mind, and vice versa, is integral to yoga, t'ai chi, and other physical arts of the East. This is why the exercise philosophy of this book unashamedly owes a great deal to these ancient practices.

With a supple and relaxed body, you will feel better physically and emotionally. The mind becomes clearer and more astute, the spirit lighter. This cannot be achieved with, for example, one hour a week of high-impact aerobics, which, while it may strengthen you, will simply bring about a short-term adrenalin buzz. To create such a delicate balance of body and spirit takes a pattern of gentle exercise, integrated into your daily life.

In the West we tend to compartmentalize our lives, creating divisions between, say, work and home, entertainment and exercise. Many Eastern philosophies, on the other hand, take a holistic view, looking at the whole person as an integrated unit. Health and happiness derive from balance in all aspects of life. Thus, paying attention to your physical and spiritual well-being is just as important as devotion to your career or your social life.

Many Eastern physical disciplines also require that you focus, concentrating totally on the task in hand, even if it is the simplest of activities, because this is the only way of releasing both body and mind from the limitations of daily life. The most basic activity, taken seriously and accomplished with complete dedication, becomes a meditation: a route to a higher understanding. Yogis will hold one *asana*, or yoga position, for a very long period of time in order

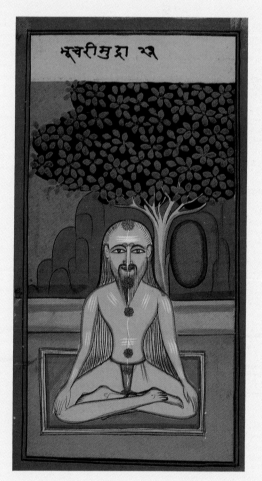

An Indian miniature painting showing the principal asana, *or posture, of Raja Yoga.*

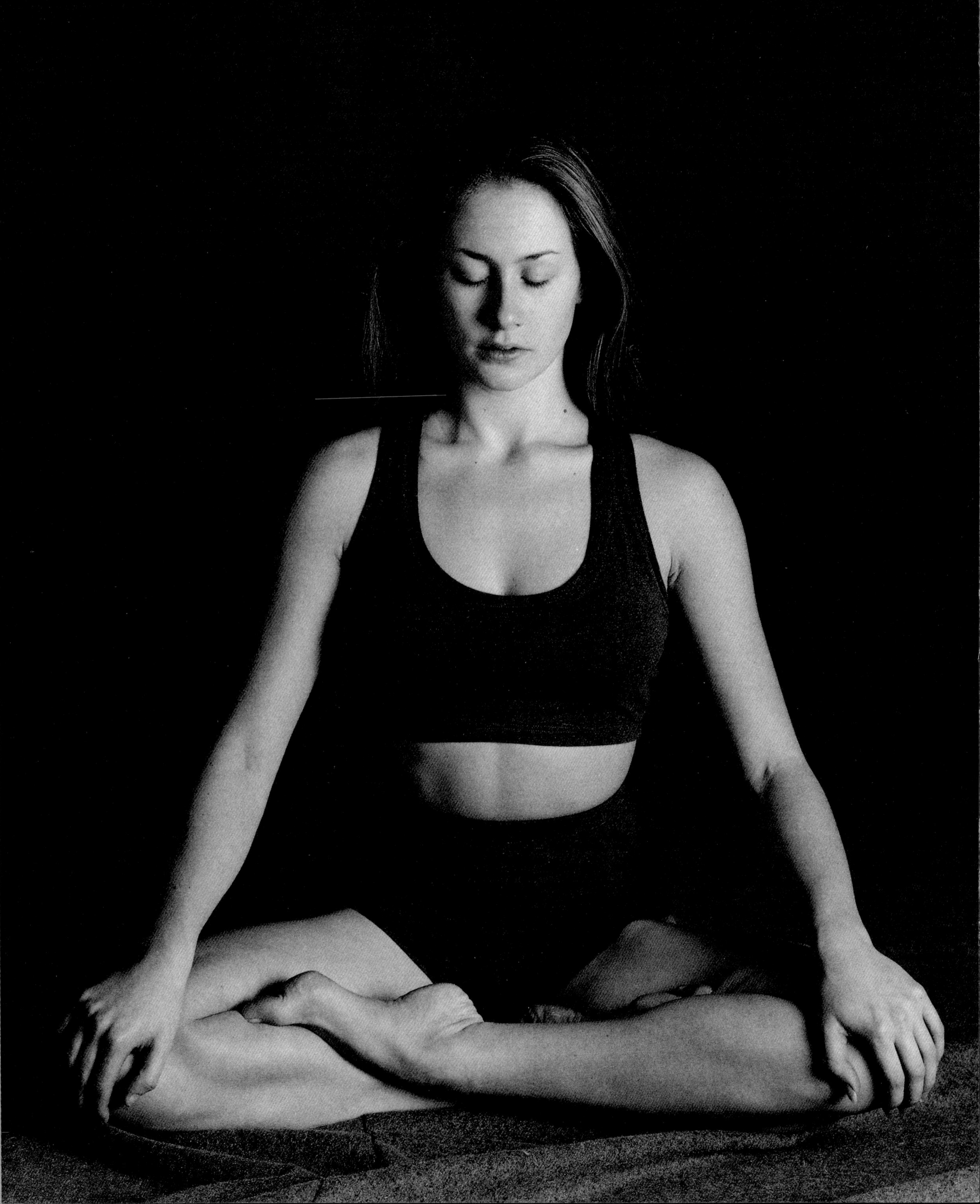

to focus their minds and their bodies. In the West, such an approach is rare: people watch TV in the gym or wear personal stereos while they run, shutting their minds to the activity they are pursuing with their bodies. This implies that physical exercise is not fulfilling enough on its own – a sad comment on the modern lifestyle.

This book advocates paying complete attention to each stretch as you do it, focusing totally on the moment. Rather than feeling bored or frustrated, you will feel happier and more centered, and your exercise will be more compelling. Each stretch will be vital in itself, rather than a means to an end.

Of course, all this is not to say that modern science cannot help us. Experts in physiotherapy, physiology, and sports medicine are constantly contributing to our understanding of the body. The way forward is to take elements from many different schools of thought and to build them into a unique and truly modern approach to health and fitness.

the method

Every day we are bombarded with images of healthy bodies. Unfortunately, we also tend to believe that we can never achieve such an ideal, attractive state. We are too old, too busy, too lazy. This book will show you that nothing is further from the truth. A busy and hectic lifestyle should not keep you from regular exercise. This book presents exercise as an integral part of daily life, rather than as a separate regime that is difficult and time-consuming to keep up. It even sets out a core series of exercises that covers all the body in only 10 minutes – short enough to fit into the busiest day. There are also exercises tailored to specific circumstances, from sitting at the desk to playing with the kids, and others that complement popular recreational sports.

Anybody, of any age, can enjoy and feel the benefits of the exercises in this book. This is not a conventional exercise program, with distinct start and end points. You are not in a competitive environment, aiming for a finishing line and striving to achieve an externally established goal. Nor do you need any special equipment or training. Rather, you are aiming to listen to your body, to understand its potential, working gently and at your own pace. This means that you are always the winner, because you can benefit immediately from the feeling of well-being that gentle stretching gives you. Achieving a suppler, healthier body is not a daunting task. When you are building a wall, you concentrate on placing each stone correctly and carefully so that soon, almost without your realizing it, the wall is in place. In the same way, as you focus on each exercise, concentrating and giving it time, your body will improve without your having to worry about it or to plan for it. Believe it or not, the process has already begun. Simply by deciding to look at this book, you are beginning to think about your health and the condition of your body. This interest is your first step.

The book presents a series of exercises organized around the part of the body they target. You can use these exercises in two ways. First, by doing each stretch carefully and paying attention to what is happening, you will learn to understand your body. At the same time, these stretches will tone your body and enhance your flexibility. You can determine the order in which you begin to explore the areas of your body and its potential. Second, the exercises can be combined into a coherent routine that will provide a thorough work-out of the whole body. This book offers a few model routines of different lengths as well as guidelines for creating your own. The important thing to realize is that the book does not teach you a few set patterns that you have to repeat endlessly, but seeks to give you the skills and the understanding to enable you to improvise on your own.

As you begin, there are a few practical considerations. Try to make your exercise as important a part of your day as any other activity. Ideally you should wear something comfortable that does not restrict your movement in any way. It does not matter what you look like, because nobody is going to see you, except perhaps a partner. The room in which you exercise should be comfortably warm. You should try as much as possible to make sure that you will not be disturbed while you are exercising. It is very frustrating to have to answer the telephone, so if you have an answering machine, switch it on.

a few words of advice

Take things gently at first, especially if you are new to exercise or returning to it after a long period. Later, as you progress, you may be tempted to remember and repeat only the stretches that come to you easily and are comfortable to do. Resist this temptation – you will only be cheating yourself. It is precisely because the other exercises require more effort that you should do them more often. Also, there is a difference between the sensation you feel when you are gently stretching muscles that are tight or unused to this kind of exercise, and the pain or discomfort that signifies an injury. Do not try to work through pain – listen carefully to your body and recognize its warning signs. If anything you feel causes you concern, you must always consult a doctor as soon as possible.

How to test your fitness

One benefit of regular gentle exercise is that it allows you to get in touch with your body, teaching you to listen to it and treat it with respect. And with this type of exercise, your own body has to be your benchmark. Your aim must be to feel better in yourself, not to reach higher or run faster than another person. That is why this book does not set guidelines for practice or regimens for improvement. Only you can determine those for yourself.

In order to do this, you have to take note of what your body is capable of and work within your own limits to try to improve whatever you want to improve.

The quick and easy test below and on pages 14–15 is a perfect place to start. It will let you know your flexibility and stamina, and encourage you to listen to your body and analyze what it tells you. In a few weeks, a month, or as often as you like, you can return to these gentle tests to check your progress. All you need is a watch, a chair, and perhaps a mirror. Above all, remember to relax and have fun – this is where your road to a healthier life begins.

Resting pulse

Every morning for three mornings, take your pulse, using your index finger, for one minute when you wake up. It is often easiest to find your pulse in your neck. Take note of your pulse each morning, then calculate the average – your resting pulse, which averages between 60 and 80 beats per minute for most people. Once you know this, you can compare it with your pulse during and after exercise. As your fitness improves, the difference will narrow.

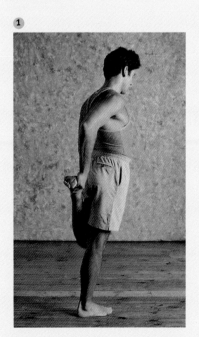

Standing thigh stretch

Stand with your feet hips' width apart. Bend your left knee and, reaching back, hold the inside of your left foot with your right hand (1). Keeping upright, pull your left foot toward your buttocks, taking care to keep your knee pointing to the floor. If you have trouble balancing, it may help to rest your free hand against the back of your chair, but remember to stay as upright as possible. Repeat on the other side.

You are aiming to touch your heel to your buttocks. Note how far away your heel is from your buttocks – this will tell you how tight your thigh muscles are.

②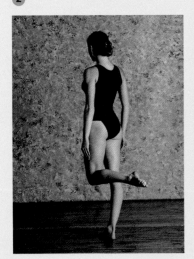

③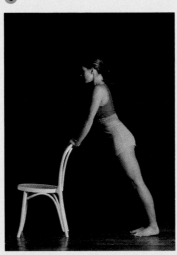

④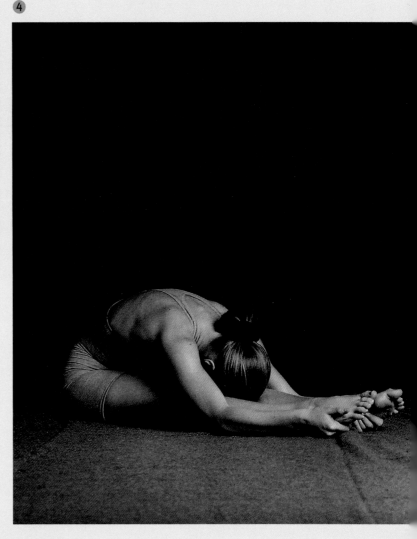

Balance

Begin by testing your balance. Clearing your mind and balancing will be the key to many of the exercises that follow, and this test can immediately tell you a lot about your balance and posture.

Stand on one leg with your arms by your sides, fixing your gaze on one point (2). You should be able to hold this for at least one minute on each leg. Note how much you are wobbling, and also whether you are steadier on one leg than on the other, as most people are.

Calf stretch

Stand about three feet from a chair, with its back toward you. Without moving your feet, lean forward and hold the back of the chair. Drop your hips, making sure that your body is as straight as possible and at a 45 degree angle to the floor (3).

Ideally, both heels should stay on the floor. If they do, then make a mental note of how tight your calf muscles feel. If your heels lift up, then note how far away from the floor they are.

Sitting forward bend, without bending your knees

Sit upright on the floor with your legs straight out in front of you and your feet flexed. Raise your arms straight up in the air above your head and reach for the ceiling to help you pull up in the lower back before bending forward from the waist. Aim to rest your hands on your toes without bending your knees (4). Once in the position, breathe and relax. Note how far toward your toes you can reach. If you find that it is very easy to touch them, try to relax more, dropping your elbows toward the floor. The distance between your hands and your feet will tell you much about the flexibility of the muscles of your back and the back of your legs.

⑤

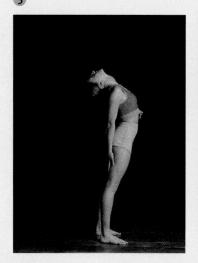
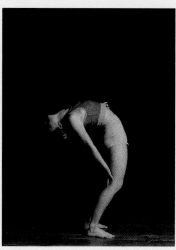

⑥

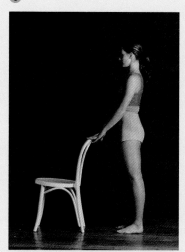

⑦

Backward bend, running hands down leg

Separate your feet a little wider than your hips for better balance, and place your hands on the backs of your thighs. Tightening your buttocks and pushing your pelvis out in front of you, bend backward, keeping your arms straight, and run your hands down your thighs (5). Note how far down your thighs your hands can go.

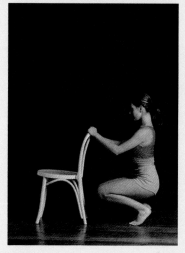

Jogging

Check your pulse before you begin, then jog in place energetically, raising your knees high, for 30 seconds (7). Check your pulse again and note the difference between the starting pulse and the finishing pulse. As your fitness improves, the difference between the pulse before and after will decrease.

Squatting, back straight, holding back of chair for support

Here is a good test for stamina, strength and balance. Stand behind your chair, resting your hands on the back for balance. Keeping your back straight and your neck long, bend your knees and sink to the floor, as low as you can go (6). Straighten your knees and return to the standing position. Repeat this as often as possible in 30 seconds. Note how many times you can complete the squat and raise sequence.

Understand your body

The human body is a miraculous construction, with an incredible range of function and movement. It relies on a complex interaction of bone, muscle, and connective tissue, motivated both involuntarily and consciously. Just raise your arm now, bending it at the elbow. Feel the biceps muscle contracting to bring the forearm bones (the radius and the ulna) toward the upper arm bone (the humerus). At the same time, you feel a stretch in the triceps muscle, which is behind the elbow and the upper arm.

This interaction, which makes the body sometimes seem so mysterious, is manifest in a number of different ways. For example, tension in your hamstring muscle can lead to back pain, because tight hamstrings can restrict movement in your pelvis, leading to stress on your back. This is why it is important to exercise with your entire body in mind, rather than focusing on so-called "problem areas," like your hips and buttocks.

The exercises in this book will encourage you to explore your body as a whole and will teach you to be as familiar with its potential as you probably already are with its limitations. To achieve this fuller understanding, it helps to have a sense of the body's overall structure. You will then be able to sense what muscles you are working when you stretch, and you will see how each action, no matter how small or apparently inconsequential, can affect your whole physique. Time taken to appreciate your body will maximize the effect of the stretches when you come to do them.

the skeleton

From a very early age we are all aware of the human skeleton. Culturally, it is a potent symbol. Yet very few people outside the medical world know much about it. It is the body's framework, to which the muscles are attached. Without the skeleton, the rest of the body would collapse. The skeleton's 206 bones account for around 20 per cent of our total body weight. Bone is living tissue, able to repair itself after breaks. It is supplied with blood and networked with nerves. Like muscles, bones can atrophy – without use, they become weaker, while bones that are used grow and remain strong.

A joint is where two bones meet, generally held together by ligaments, which is the connective tissue. At a joint, each bone is covered in cartilage, which is strong and slippery. Each type of joint is suited to a specific type of motion. A "ball and socket" joint, like the shoulder, is designed for rotational motion. The hip is also a ball and socket joint, but it is designed for a far more limited range of movement than the shoulder. "Hinge" joints, like the elbow, are

the bones of the body

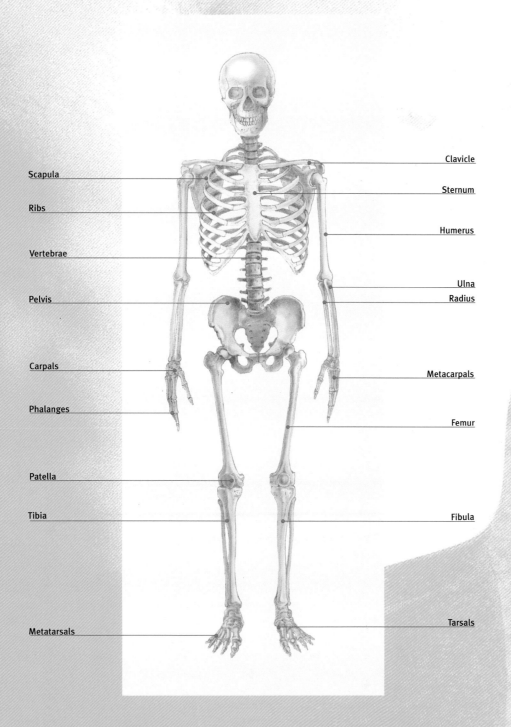

Scapula

Ribs

Vertebrae

Pelvis

Carpals

Phalanges

Patella

Tibia

Metatarsals

Clavicle

Sternum

Humerus

Ulna

Radius

Metacarpals

Femur

Fibula

Tarsals

designed for backward and forward movement. "Pivot" joints link, for example, the 24 vertebrae allowing them to glide and twist. "Gliding" joints, like the ankle, allow one bone to slide across the others. The condition of the joints is an important factor in our flexibility. If they are underused they can stiffen, but if they are used to their full potential, the ligaments become more flexible, and their range of movement can be maximized – something you will become increasingly aware of as you improve your body.

the muscles

The body has about 600 different muscles, accounting for around one half of our total body weight. Muscle tissue is highly specialized. There are "involuntary" muscles, such as those that make your organs function, over which we do not really have conscious control, and "voluntary" muscles, which are generally those attached to bones and generate motion. There is also cardiac muscle in the heart, which is not under conscious control either. Voluntary muscles can act in only one way – they contract. Once the contraction ends, they "pay out," or lengthen, to their resting position. You cannot order your muscles to relax, only "not to contract." This means that relaxation is really a state of doing nothing at all (see pages 20–27).

Because of this, muscles are often organized in pairs, called "antagonists," around joints. A "flexor" bends a joint, while an "extensor" straightens it. When one muscle in the pair contracts to make a movement, the other must be in a relaxed state. In bending your elbow, one muscle, the biceps, contracts to raise your arm, while the triceps is relaxed; then the triceps contracts to straighten it, while the biceps relaxes slowly.

Muscles are under the control of the nervous system. In simple terms, your brain sends a command to a muscle to act in a certain way. At the same time, the brain always tries to protect the body. A reflex designed to prevent overstretching forces a muscle to contract if it is stretched too quickly and violently. But if you gently move into the stretch, this reflex is not called into action, so you are able to achieve a deeper stretch without working against your body. By the same token, bouncing during an exercise only activates the protective reflex, cause muscles to contract rather than stretch deeper.

Voluntary muscles, however, are there to be used. Well-used muscles develop in strength and size, while unused muscles, like the bones they surround, atrophy, or decrease in strength and size. And of course the only way to help your muscles develop is through regular exercise.

the muscles of the body

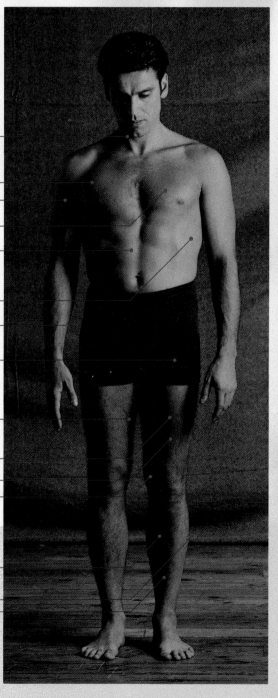

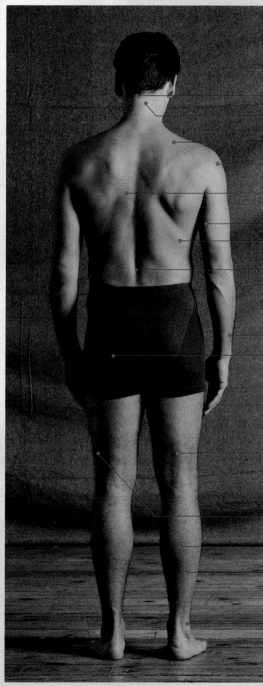

Sternolleido Mastodeus

Pectoralis Minor

Biceps

Pectoralis Major

Rectus Abdominus

External Abdominal

Flexors of Arm and Hand

Iliopsoas

Adductors

Vastus Literalis

Rectus Femoris

Vastus Medialis

Tibialis Anterior

Peroneus Extensor

Semispinalis Capitis

Splenius Capitis

Trapezius

Deltoid

Rhomboid

Triceps

Latissimus Dorsi

Erectors

Hand Extensors

Gluteus

Hamstrings

Iliotibial Tract

Gastrocnemius

Soleus

Achilles Tendon

Relaxation

Relaxation – doing nothing, simply letting your mind and body find a natural and calm state – does not come easily to many of us. It is difficult to leave the stresses of daily life behind us, even for a few minutes. There are techniques, however, to release our thoughts and center ourselves. A relaxed state enhances the effectiveness and pleasure of any exercise.

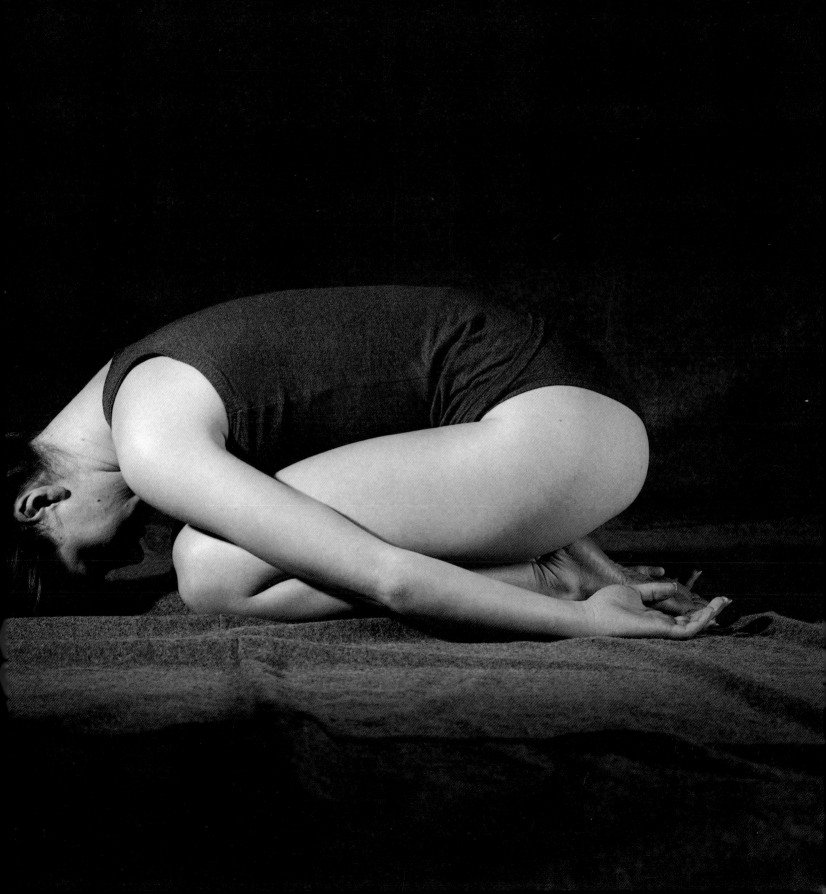

Relaxation

For a fit and healthy life, everything must be balanced: the mind should be calm yet alert; the breathing free and easy; the muscles strong yet relaxed; the joints free to use their full range of movement. A tiger at rest is calm and relaxed, but you know that it has the capacity for great strength and power.

You might be surprised to see a chapter on relaxation in an exercise book. It would be more relevant and more useful to wonder why the need for relaxation is so often ignored in modern fitness and health programs, especially since it has become increasingly clear that we must relax and conquer stress to function at the peak of our abilities.

It used to be fashionable to believe that the only way to improve your body was to push it to the limit. You ignored what the brain was telling you and stretched that much further, jumped that much higher, tried that much harder, until your pulse was racing and you could not do any more. Think how often you have been to a gym and seen someone with their body clenched, sweat pouring down their face, and the veins popping out of their necks, trying to force their body to be fitter. Pushing the body to the brink can lead to serious injury and will never allow the body to reveal its true potential.

Think for a moment of somebody you admire. It might be an athlete in peak physical condition, a dancer, or even a colleague who always seems in command of the situation. What these people have in common is that they achieve great feats of strength, beauty, and organization from a state of centered calmness. The Olympic athlete at the start of the race is physically relaxed and mentally alert. The athlete allows his or her body to perform at its maximum by freeing it from stress and letting the muscles respond freely in the way they have been trained. If you want to improve your fitness in the same way, you must examine this relationship between mind and body.

Now, take a moment to stop reading and sit quietly observing your body. As you sit here, your physical body – the combination of muscles, bones, connective tissue, organs, nerves, and so on – is in varying states of relaxation and tension. A certain amount of tension is required to keep the body upright, but beyond that, external circumstances, as well as your state of mind, can effect your physical state. Is the room too cold? Is your waistband a little tight? Are you in a hurry? Have you been having a bad day? Are you concerned about a meeting later in the day or later in the week? All these factors can effect your physical state, creating tension, inhibiting flexibility, and hindering the development of a fit and healthy body.

Of course, relaxation on its own is certainly not going to make you fit. It is only one part of a total fitness plan. You must also stretch and exercise

You should always take a few minutes both before and after your regular exercise practice to relax or recuperate. The time you spend beforehand will help you concentrate on the task in hand; afterward, the few minutes of calm and relaxation will allow your mind and body to benefit fully from the exercise experience.

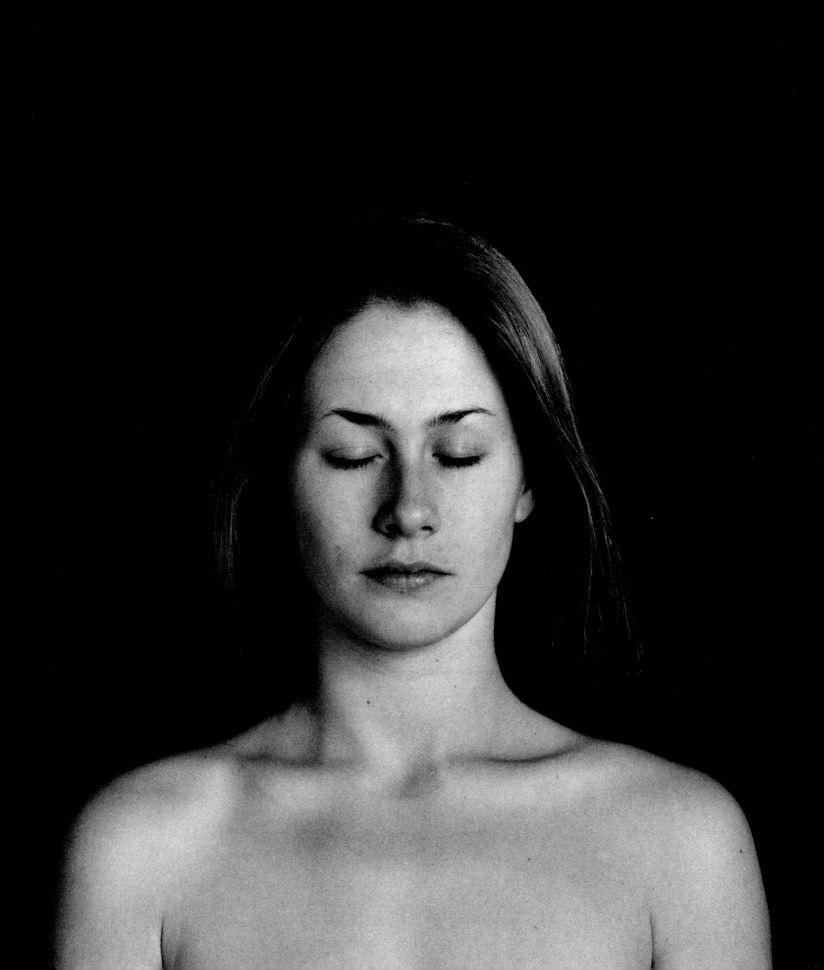

regularly, and if you want to play demanding sports, you have to develop additional stamina and strength. Relaxation plays a crucial role in all of this.

Exercise itself can help you to relax. In order to get the maximum benefit from the gentle stretches explained in this book, it is important to concentrate completely on your body. You will find that, as you focus on the exercises and your body's response to them, day-to-day mental stresses will recede from your mind. In the same way, Zen monks rake their pebble gardens into regular, prescribed patterns, using the work as a physical meditation.

Most people have experienced the sensation of calmness and optimism that follows exercise but have never drawn the natural conclusions from it. If exercise makes your body feel relaxed and peaceful, shouldn't that same mental state be used to achieve better results – and have a better time – during exercise? If you consciously relax before you exercise, clearing your mind and your body of the stresses that have accumulated during your day-to-day life, you will not have to waste time and energy as you exercise to break through that residual tension. This will enhance the effectiveness of your exercise, allowing you to benefit fully and enjoy yourself even more.

The exercises that follow will help you to achieve the relaxed state that will enable you to stretch further and work out better. You should always take a few minutes both before and after your regular exercise practice to relax or recuperate. The time you spend beforehand will help you concentrate on the task in hand, ridding your mind of all other daily concerns; afterward, the few minutes of calm and relaxation will allow your mind and body to benefit fully from the exercise experience, as you bathe in tranquillity and peace.

But you do not need to restrict these simple relaxation techniques to your exercise practice. A few minutes' mental escape from the concerns of everyday life, clearing your mind, is beneficial in any circumstances. Treat yourself – you will be amazed by the results.

full body guided relaxation

Find a quiet, warm room where you will not be disturbed. You may want to take the phone off the hook or put the answering machine on. It is essential that external circumstances will not interrupt you.

Lie on your back on the floor with your legs stretched out and your arms by your sides. Turn your palms face up. Make sure you are comfortable. You may

A certain amount of tension is required to keep the body upright, but beyond that, external circumstances, as well as your state of mind, can affect your physical state, creating excess tension and inhibiting flexibility. However, relaxation is only one part of a total fitness plan. You must also stretch and exercise regularly.

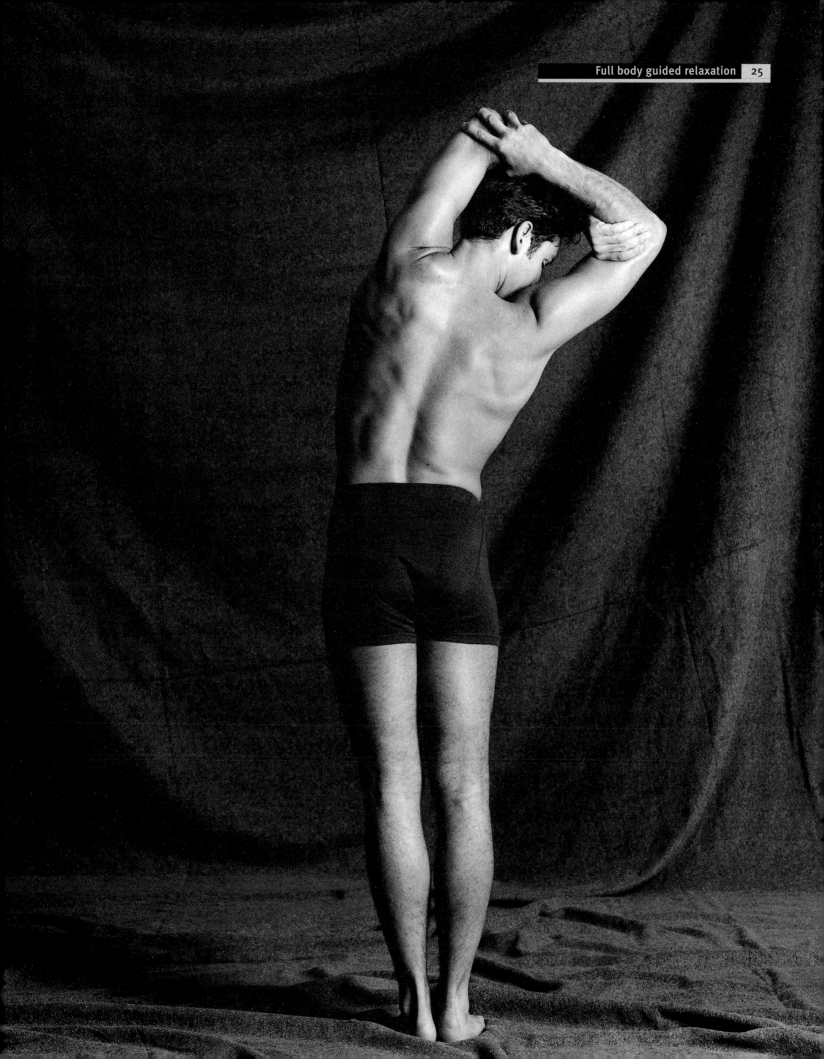

wish to rest the back of your head on a book or a pillow, or cover yourself with a blanket if you are chilly. Closing your eyes, breathe deeply. Start to visualize the parts of your body. Begin by concentrating mentally on your feet and ankles. Flex your feet and tighten them as much as you can. Hold for a moment and then "let go," allowing them to relax totally. Repeat this two more times. Now you know your feet are completely relaxed. Move your attention to the legs and knees. Tighten your legs and knees as much as you can, pushing them down into the floor, and hold for a couple of seconds before "letting go." Repeat this twice more, and then your legs and knees will be totally relaxed.

Continue working through every part of your body. Tighten and release the hips and buttocks, tummy, upper chest, the upper, middle and lower back, the shoulders, arms, hands, and even your face. You should not ignore any part of your body. When you have completed this process, your whole body should feel relaxed and heavy. It is not very likely that you will want to move at this point, but if you feel at all uncomfortable, make the necessary gentle adjustments to your position.

Now mentally return to your feet. Without doing anything physically, check that you are not holding on to any unnecessary tension. If you find that you are, concentrate for a moment on freeing yourself of that tension. Move through your body, running this mental check.

By now your whole body should be totally relaxed. Breathing naturally, stay in this relaxed position for at least 10 minutes. Finish by opening your eyes and stretching slowly.

Make sure that you do not rush into your next activity. If you try to get up too quickly, you will feel very faint and dizzy. However, if you come to at a slow and natural pace, you will feel calm, invigorated, and more than capable of taking on whatever the world may choose to throw at you.

relaxation exercises

If you do not have time for the full body guided relaxation, there are several techniques that can be done either standing or sitting and can seamlessly be incorporated into your warm-up, or into the pattern of your day-to-day life.

One of the simplest exercises uses your breath to help you to relax. Simply stand with your feet hips' width apart, keeping your knees slightly bent, or sit upright on a firm chair. As you breathe out, think of your shoulders being relaxed and your whole body loose. A lot of tension and stress is held in the neck and shoulder area. A number of simple stretches can quickly relieve some of that tension.

Shrug (see page 137)
As you breathe in, raise your shoulders up toward your ears as high as you can. Hold them there for five seconds, then, as you exhale, let them drop freely. Relax, breathing in, then as you breathe out, try to relax your shoulders and arms a little more — there may not be any visible movement, but you will feel an internal release.

Shoulder rolls (see page 44)
Standing, with your arms relaxed by your sides, raise one shoulder up to your ear, then rotate it slowly forward then down, then draw it back and up again toward your ear, keeping the movement as full and as circular as you can. Do this three times in one direction, then reverse for three times, before changing to the other side. Pay attention to keep the rest of your body as still as possible without tensing, leaving the movement to your shoulders.

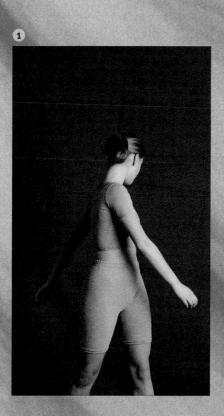
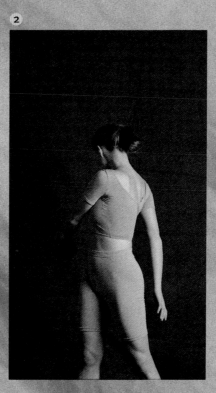

Playground swing
Stand with your feet hips' width apart. Relax the knees and let your arms hang free. Moving freely from the hips, twist your upper body to the left, allowing your right arm to swing in front of you and your left arm to swing behind your back (1). Then swing to the right, reversing the arms (2). Continue to swing in this way for at least five minutes, keeping your neck and shoulders relaxed and your arms free.

You can also swing your arms backward and forward from your shoulders, again keeping the rest of your body relaxed and your movements free and easy. If you feel that you need to free your shoulders more, try circling your arms. You might have seen swimmers doing this as the warm up for a big race. Standing firmly with your right foot about a step in front of the left, let your left arm swing freely backward and forward for a moment. Use the forward momentum to swing your arm up and over so that it traces a complete circle. Repeat as often as you like.

Breathing

This chapter aims to encourage you to be aware of your breathing and to understand how learning to work with your full breath can help you both during exercise and throughout your day-to-day life. With regular practice you will begin to free up your breathing, allowing your body to work naturally without tension, and giving you the ability to exercise more freely and effectively.

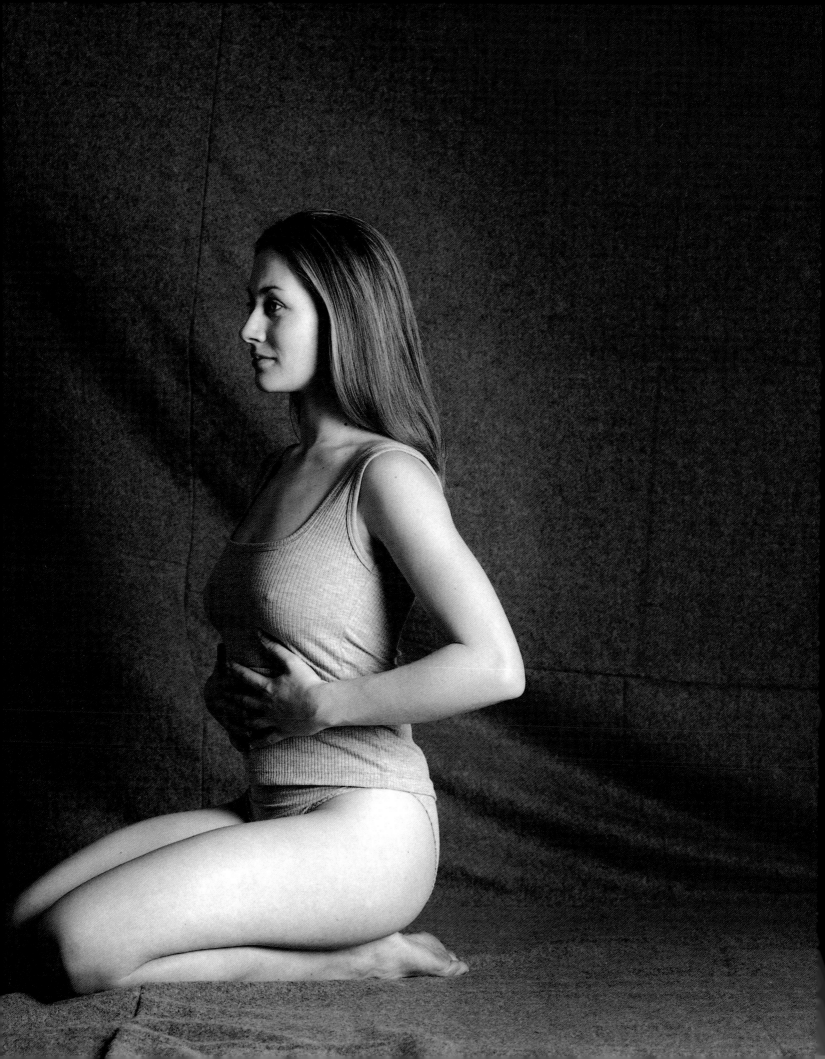

Breathing

Think about this: the volume of our daily intake of air is five times more than our daily food and fluid intake combined. The "breath of life" is as vital to us as the water we drink and the food we eat, yet because we are surrounded by the air that we breathe in normal day-to-day life, we do not really notice our breathing. Most of us care less about the quality of the air we breathe than about the quality of our food and drink.

The body breathes automatically – it is not possible to decide consciously to stop breathing, because the body will eventually force the next breath to occur. However, the combination of bad habits and day-to-day stresses can restrict the natural flow of our breath just as they can restrict our natural freedom of movement.

The breath and emotions are interrelated. When you are angry, you might hold your breath, or, if you are particularly nervous or stressed, your breathing might become very short and shallow. Most people only use their lungs to their maximum potential when they laugh or cry deeply. And laughter and crying both leave behind a feeling of relaxation, a release of emotional tension. Think of how tired and cleansed you feel after a bout of wholehearted laughter, or the relief you feel after a deep sigh.

Breathing is also related to feelings of physical tension or stress in the body. If you have ever had a massage, you will have noticed that as your muscles relax, your breathing deepens and slows. It is not surprising then that you can use your breathing during exercise to help release your muscles, thus enhancing the effectiveness of your stretching.

This is by no means a modern idea. In the ancient practices of yoga or t'ai chi, for example, instructions on how to breathe are woven into the exercise instructions. Similarly, the 19th-century actor F. M. Alexander, in attempting to cure his loss of voice, realized that the breath and the body are interlinked. His "Alexander Technique" for improving posture and breathing is finding more and more 20th-century followers.

By working with your breath as well as your body, you will begin to free up your breathing, allowing your body to work naturally. With regular practice, it won't be long before your breathing will become easier and deeper, and this will have a major effect on the quality of your life. You might find that you don't feel like you are rushing as much as you once did, or perhaps you can deal with stressful situations more easily. You may find that you simply feel a little lighter and more content. But at the very least, by harnessing your breathing, you will be able to exercise more productively, and that can only be for the best.

the breathing mechanism

Breathing is the most natural thing in the world. It is at the very center of our physical lives. It is instinctive and involuntary and yet how often do you let it work naturally? Most people most of the time are unconsciously hindering the full extent of their breath. To find out how much we are holding on, we must take a moment to think about how the breathing mechanism works.

In very basic physiological terms, our breathing system is a series of pipes and sacks that provides a large surface area for the exchange of gases. Basically, we breathe in oxygen and breathe out carbon dioxide (CO_2) as well as other waste products.

As you breathe in through your mouth or your nostrils, the air travels along the windpipe (which includes the larynx, where the vocal chords are) and down into the lungs.

The lungs themselves have no muscles. They react to changes in the size of the thoracic cavity (the area of chest containing the lungs) created by the diaphragm, the intercostal muscles (those between the ribs), and a neck muscle. The change in the size of the thoracic cavity creates a change in pressure internally. When the diaphragm flattens and the intercostal muscles cause the chest to expand, the lungs take in air because internal pressure is lower than atmospheric pressure. During exhalation, the diaphragm and the intercostal muscles relax, and the volume of the thoracic cavity decreases.

Breathing is totally involuntary: you cannot choose to hold your breath indefinitely, because ultimately you will black out, and as soon as you do, your body will begin to breathe again. The breathing mechanism is regulated by the level of CO_2 in the blood. Once it exceeds a certain level, the brain demands a new breath.

The maximum volume of air that can move in and out of the lungs is called their "vital capacity." During normal, resting breathing, the average person only exchanges around 10 per cent of the total air in the lungs (approximately one pint, or 600 ml). After a normal, resting exhalation, you could exhale an additional amount of around five pints (3 litres). This is because the lungs have a far greater capacity than we use in ordinary breathing. Conscious deep breathing allows us to exchange about 80 per cent of the air in the lungs with each breath. The remaining 20 per cent is called "residual air" and remains in the lungs at all times.

This is the process that begins when you are born and stops when you die, and it is much simpler than it sounds. It is only mentioned here because many of us make it complicated. Look at the breathing of a young child, and you will see the whole system working effortlessly. All the movement is centered in the middle of the body. This is because that child has not had time to learn any bad habits that can interfere with the natural process.

Now take a moment to observe yourself. Is your head freely balanced on the top of the spine, or is it held tightly in position? Is your jaw or throat tense? Are your shoulders braced up toward your ears or slumped forward? Is the upper chest caving in or being pulled up? Is your stomach relaxed? How free are your knees and feet? All these little details, habits born from experience, can effect your breathing, making it inefficient. If your posture is bad, for example, the muscles that create the changes in the body that lead to the intake and outflow of breath are restricted in their natural movement, and the lungs cannot expand to their full potential. This can result in breathing only in our upper ribs, a habit we get used to and accept as the norm.

The most important thing, however, is not to worry. There is no right way to breathe, only bad habits that can get in the way of optimal breathing.

breathing exercises

Exercise increases the body's demand for oxygen. This is why you breathe faster and deeper, especially during aerobic exercise like swimming or running. Probably you have noticed that you continue to breath deeply for a few minutes after you stop exercising. This deep breathing helps the body to recover from its exertions.

Although the exercises in this book are not aerobic exercises, breathing is still an important part of gentle stretching. Your body is still working hard, and will have an increased demand for oxygen, which you can supply by breathing deeply and fully before, during, and after your stretches.

Your breath is a barometer of how difficult you find the exercises. You should aim to keep your breathing deep and natural throughout your workouts, but if you suddenly have to gasp for breath or blow the breath out vigorously through your mouth, then this is a good sign that you might be pushing the stretch too far and risking injury. When you are holding a new and challenging position, your instinct may be to panic a little when this happens, which results in shallow breathing or, worse still, holding the breath

Although the exercises in this book are not aerobic exercises, breathing is still an important component in gentle stretching. Your body is still working hard, and thus will have an increased demand for oxygen, which you can supply by breathing deeply and fully before, during, and after your stretches.

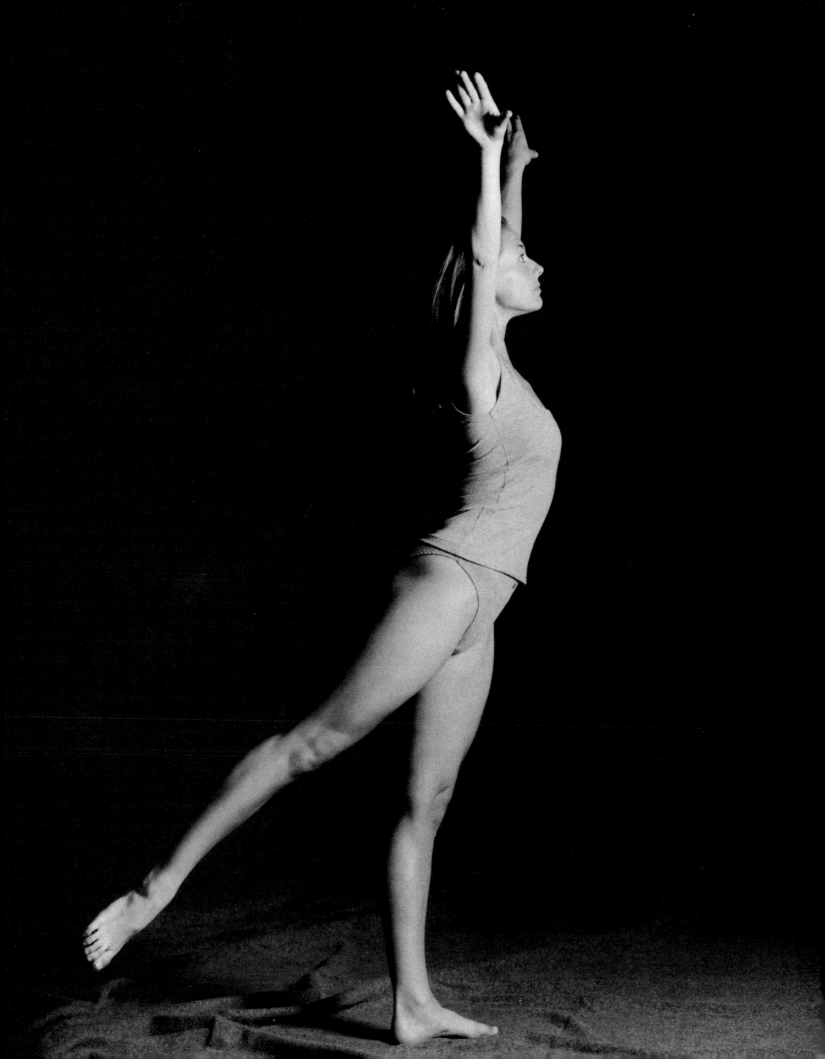

altogether. At these times tell yourself to breathe naturally – you will find that the exercise becomes much easier, and you will feel calmer. As you work your way through the book, the descriptions of the exercises will often suggest that you "breathe through" a stretch. This means exactly what has been described above: that you should consciously use your breathing to help you to relax your muscles.

Unless you are doing a specific exercise that suggests you should do otherwise, breathe through your nose at all times. It is more relaxing, and the whole object is to relax and enjoy yourself. If you spend a few minutes concentrating on your breathing before or after you exercise, it will help you to relax, improving your posture, centering your thoughts, and making your exercise much more productive.

These simple exercises are ideal for incorporating into your warm-up program. Keep in mind that they are only a means to an end, and that end is relaxation. Unless you have a job that requires a lot of public speaking (like teaching, acting, or politics), you do not need to be too concerned with the breathing process.

Because of the calming effects of breathing exercises, you can use them any time and any place. If you find yourself in a stressful situation, the wave breath can help you relax, without anybody noticing that you are doing it. It can also help you stop smoking. The deep breathing can help you to conquer your craving for cigarettes in two ways. You are replacing one activity – smoking – with another, harmless activity – breathing – and the required concentration on your breath helps you focus on something other than your desire for a cigarette.

Relax and enjoy the time these exercises allow you. Remember, there is no right way to breathe, only lots of ways to interfere with nature's process. If you ever feel that you are getting too serious, then take a moment to think about something completely different.

The whispered "Ah"

This exercise from the Alexander Technique is a great way of becoming aware of your breath. It can be done either standing or sitting, but it is probably better if you stand. First find a comfortably warm, quiet room and make sure that you won't be disturbed. Stand in the middle of the room and if you have a window, face toward it so you can look out. Looking at a view will help you to relax and keep you from over-concentrating on the exercise. To start, do not do anything physically – instead, mentally scan your body with the following checklist in mind:

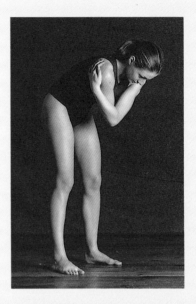

The hug

This exercise will allow you to feel how deeply you can breathe. Stand upright with your feet hips' width apart. Cross your arms in front of you, and rest the palms of your hands on your shoulders. It should look as if you were giving youself a hug. In this position, relax your arms and shoulders. There should be no unnecessary tension in the upper body. Drop your head forward, bending from the waist. Breathe all the way out, then slowly, naturally allow a big breath in. You will be aware of your ribs opening in your back, and it should feel like the breath will be moving right down your spine. This is very good for relaxing the lower back, if nothing else. Repeat a few times. Drop your arms, then return to an upright position, slowly – if you stand up too quickly you will become dizzy.

- Your weight should be evenly balanced over your feet, your ankles free.
- Your knees should be relaxed and not locked.
- Your hips should be relaxed, your pelvis dropped freely toward the floor.
- Your tummy muscles should be relaxed.
- Your shoulders should be dropped and your arms hanging free.
- Your neck should be relaxed. This can be done by dropping your nose very slightly and imagining your head floating toward the ceiling.

Once you have made your observations, let your jaw drop open, with your tongue resting lightly behind your lower teeth. Think of something nice and smile a little. Now, breathe out gently on a whispered *Ah*, until you have run out of air. There should be very little sound. If you hear a rattling in the throat or any vocalized sound, you are probably holding onto some tension.

Close your mouth. Instead of immediately breathing in, think of doing nothing, and you will find that the ribs spring out of their own accord. Remember that if you concentrate on breathing out correctly, then breathing in will be automatic and easy. Repeat this process five times before resting and clearing your mind altogether. Do not be surprised if you feel a little dizzy. If you do, stop for a moment before continuing.

The wave

The next breathing exercise, using vizualization, is a very good way of letting the breath relax you, centering your thoughts and preparing you for exercise. Lie on your back on the floor, with your legs straight and your arms by your sides, palms up. Close your eyes. Your mouth is closed, but your jaw hangs loose, and your teeth should not be clenched. Relax your tongue.

Breathe in deeply, feeling your belly expanding like a balloon, for a count of three. Hold the breath for a count of three, before exhaling through your nose for the count of three. Repeat this, concentrating fully on your breathing, keeping your upper body free of tension. As you continue breathing like this, you will find that you fall into your own natural rhythm. Some people may find it more satisfying to breathe to the count of four or maybe even five. Once you find your natural rhythm, you will be able to visualize a pattern to the breath much like a wave rolling up the beach.

As you breathe in, feel the breath fill your belly first, then move up to fill your middle chest, your ribs expanding, then higher to fill your upper chest, perhaps even causing your shoulders to rise slightly. As you breathe out, feel it reversing – as it leaves your upper chest, your shoulders relax; as it leaves your middle chest, your ribs relax; and as it leaves your belly, it sinks. Repeat for as long as you wish.

Targeted exercises

By concentrating on each area of
your body individually, you will
come to understand your
physicality, how it functions and
how your muscles interrelate. You
will be able to spend more time
on those areas of your body in
which you feel most tension or
that otherwise need most care.

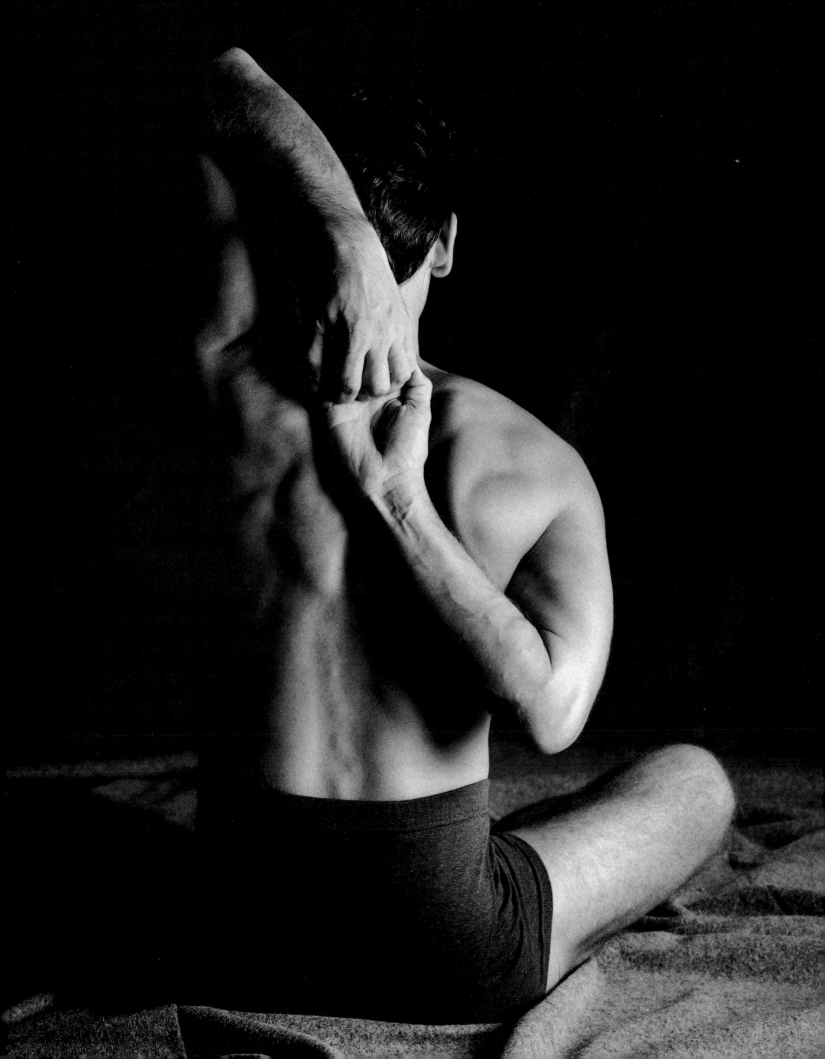

Targeted exercises
general advice

In order to strengthen and improve your body, you must first learn to observe how its different components work by concentrating on each part separately – just as mechanics must strip an engine before they can really understand how it functions.

The following chapters will help you in this exploration, suggesting key exercises for each part of the body. You can work in logical order if you wish, beginning with the head and working down, or beginning with the feet and working up, or you can just dive in and begin wherever you feel like.

Especially when you are just beginning, try to use the exercises to help you locate and pinpoint exactly which muscle works where and when. Relax into each position and observe how your body feels within it. Try to understand the ways in which the muscles work together. You will find that some exercises appear in more than one section. This is because they work more than one part of the body. These can be useful if you want quick, multipurpose stretches when you might not have that much time.

Only once you are familiar with the exercises and your body is becoming stronger and suppler should you begin to increase the number of repetitions, to hold a position for longer, or to move to more advanced variations. Of course, each person's body is different and you may find that one area is naturally very flexible while another may be very tense. As you work through the following sections you should note your personal areas of tension, so you can build your future routines around your personal needs.

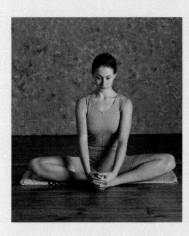

Hips and buttocks, page 70

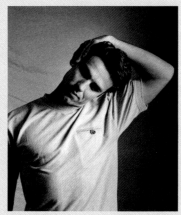

Neck, page 42

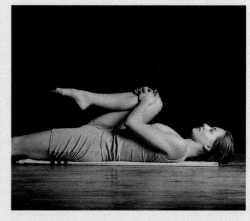

Back, page 52

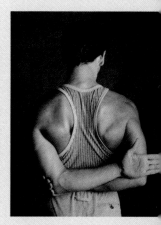

Shoulders, page 44

The most important aspect of exercise is listening to your body. Do not do anything that you are uncomfortable with. You will achieve more by relaxing and working at a gentle pace than you will by pushing yourself too hard.

1 Before you exercise, you should spend a few minutes clearing your mind, breathing deeply, and consciously relaxing before you start.

2 You must always begin by working very gently and slowly, releasing any tension throughout your body, before you move to more advanced stretches.

3 The warm-up is an essential part of your exercise session. The first two or three exercises in each section are best for warming up that part of the body. Used in combination they will gently work you from top to toe.

4 It is important to have a "cool-down" after any period of exercise. Just as you begin slowly, you should slow down gently, rather than stopping abruptly.

5 After exercising, try taking a few minutes consciously relaxing your mind and body. Enjoy a little tranquility before moving to the next activity of your day.

Face
targeted exercises

The old adage that we should smile because it takes fewer muscles to smile than to frown neatly shows our instinctive awareness that our face is manipulated by a sophisticated group of muscles. Working and toning these muscles will achieve greater freedom of movement in our faces, and also moderate the gradual sagging that comes with age.

If we keep the facial muscles strong and supportive, our faces will remain firmer. Also, gentle exercise of those muscles will improve circulation, helping to keep the skin glowing. It is best to learn the following exercises in front of a mirror. They will probably make you laugh at first as you make faces like you did as a child. But, as they say, laughter is the best medicine, so feel free.

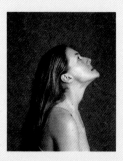

Chin to ceiling
Sitting or standing comfortably, tilt your head backward, lifting your chin toward the ceiling. This may result in your bottom teeth moving in front of your top teeth for the duration of the stretch. You should feel this in the bottom of your chin and through your neck.

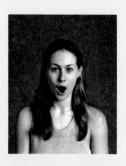

"Ow"
Say "ow" very slowly and carefully, starting with your mouth wide open in a big circle and working it quite strongly throughout, until, at the final "w" sound, your mouth is nearly closed. Repeat this as many times as feels comfortable.

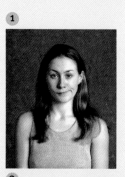
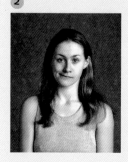

Alternate smiles
Keeping the right side of your face still, stretch the left side of your mouth toward your ear (1), then reverse (2). You will feel the stretch in your face as well as your neck. If this is easier on one side, practice by holding one side of your face as you stretch the other, so the muscles can learn the pattern of movement.

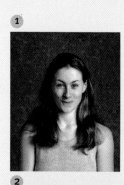
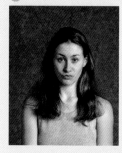

Purse, pig, and grimace
Begin by pursing your mouth, pulling your lips together as tightly as possible (1). Then, keeping your lips together, unclench them and push them forward as far as they will go in the shape of a pig's snout (2). Then pull your mouth as wide as it will go, as if the corners could reach your ears. Repeat five times.

Forehead stretch
Raise and lower your eyebrows in the manner of Groucho Marx. As you do this, you will feel a strong stretch running from your forehead down through your ears – in fact, your ears may even wiggle a little. You can repeat the stretch as many times as feels comfortable.

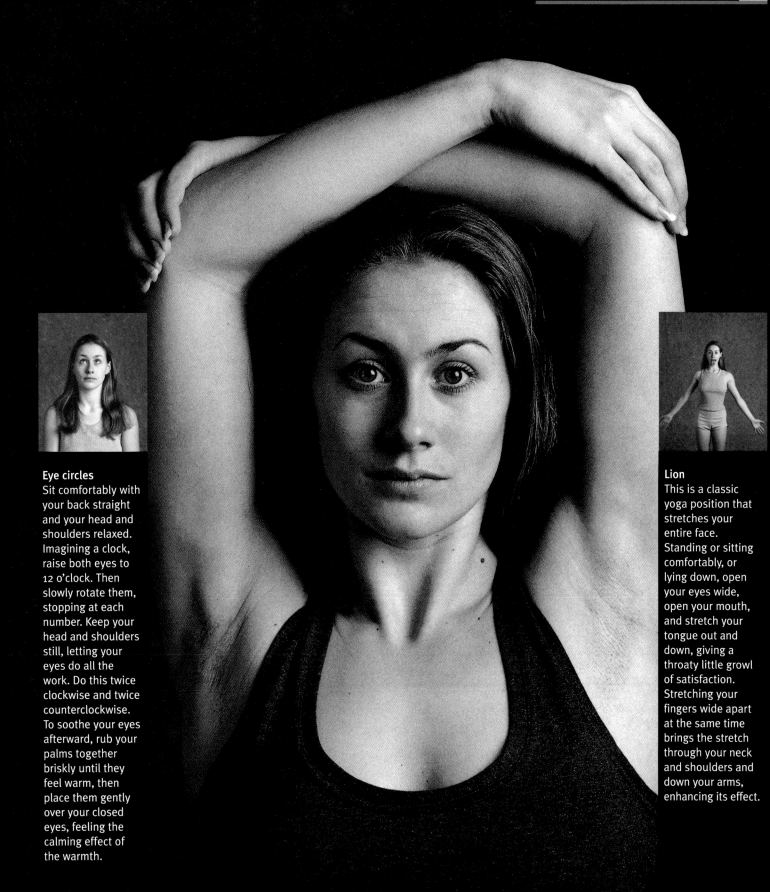

Eye circles
Sit comfortably with your back straight and your head and shoulders relaxed. Imagining a clock, raise both eyes to 12 o'clock. Then slowly rotate them, stopping at each number. Keep your head and shoulders still, letting your eyes do all the work. Do this twice clockwise and twice counterclockwise. To soothe your eyes afterward, rub your palms together briskly until they feel warm, then place them gently over your closed eyes, feeling the calming effect of the warmth.

Lion
This is a classic yoga position that stretches your entire face. Standing or sitting comfortably, or lying down, open your eyes wide, open your mouth, and stretch your tongue out and down, giving a throaty little growl of satisfaction. Stretching your fingers wide apart at the same time brings the stretch through your neck and shoulders and down your arms, enhancing its effect.

Neck targeted exercises

There are few better examples of the beauty and complexity of the human body than the neck. Acting essentially as the junction of the head and the torso, the neck not only bridges the vital gap between the brain and the body, channeling the spinal column, but it also has the potential for a huge range of movement. It can rotate the head 90 degrees left and right or tilt it back and forth, and any combination of the two. At the same time, the neck carries a very heavy burden – your head, which accounts for around 14–18 lbs (6–8 kgs) of your total body weight.

Initially, neck stretches can be quite uncomfortable, which may seem worrying. But if you work gently to begin with, paying attention to the messages your body is sending, you do not need to be frightened of letting your head go. It will not take long to feel the benefits of an increased range of movement in your neck.

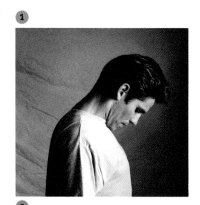

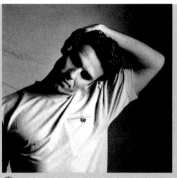

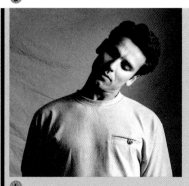

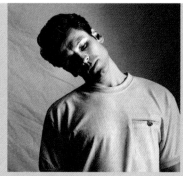

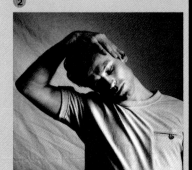

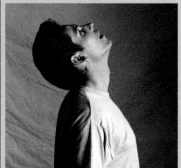

Sideways head clasp
Sitting comfortably on the floor or in a chair, tilt your head to the left, so your left ear approaches your shoulder. Reach up with your left arm and hold your head (1). Relax your left arm so its weight exerts a natural, gentle pull. To enhance this stretch, lift your right arm until it is horizontal and flex your hand at the wrist. Hold for 20 seconds, then release and switch sides (2).

Head cross
Drop your head forward until your chin is on your chest (1). Slowly raise it, then lower it to the right, aiming to touch the ear to the shoulder (2). Then lower your head to the left, again aiming to touch your ear to your shoulder (3). Finally, look up toward the ceiling. Keep your shoulders still and level and let your jaw hang loose (4). Do this sequence three times.

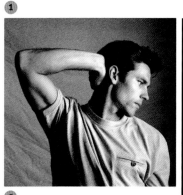

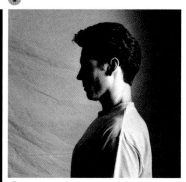

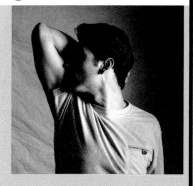

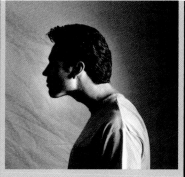

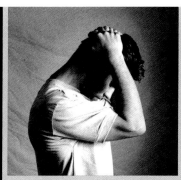

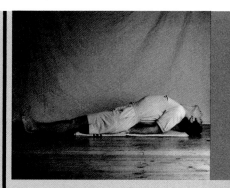

Head and neck twist

Sit comfortably, either in a chair or on the floor. Place your right hand on the back of your head, at the base of your skull. Tilt your head down and turn to look toward your left shoulder, using your hand to push your head lightly (1). Then turn your head, looking up and to the right, pushing your head against your right arm (2). Reverse. Try to hold each of the positions for at least 15 seconds.

Hen

It helps to visualize this movement by thinking about the comical way a chicken moves its head. Tuck your chin down, without dropping your neck forward, then draw it back slowly (1), keeping your back and shoulders as still as possible. Then slowly draw your head forward, leading from the chin, until it is stretched as far in front as possible (2). Repeat this movement five or six times.

Head clasp

This is a very good stretch for curing headaches. Standing or sitting, drop your head forward, bringing your chin toward your chest, but keeping your back straight. Clasp your hands behind the back of your head. Relax your arms, allowing their weight to pull your head gently inward and downward. Hold on to this position for at least 10 seconds, then release and relax.

Fish

This is a yoga exercise that is very good for the neck. Lie on your back with your palms down, arms under your buttocks. Supporting your weight on your elbows, lift your upper body, arching your back until the top of your head rests on the floor. Remember to keep your weight on your elbows and your back arched but relaxed. Breathe deeply, feeling your chest opening and your lungs expanding. Hold for 30 seconds to a minute before lowering yourself carefully.

Shoulders
targeted exercises

Your shoulders are the first area of the body to suffer when the stresses and strains of everyday living impose on your physical well-being. One of the first signs of tension or stress is that our shoulders rise toward our ears, and it takes a considerable time and effort to release them.

Shoulders can also suffer for simpler, physical reasons, such as carrying a heavy shoulder bag or sitting awkwardly: just leaning on the armrests of a chair can push your shoulders up. As you learn to relax and release your shoulders, your posture will improve, your breath become deeper, and you will feel more at ease.

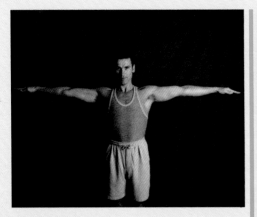

"T" shape
Standing comfortably, slowly raise your arms, keeping them straight at the elbows, until they are horizontal to the floor. Extend them fully, stretching your fingers out, at the same time making sure you do not raise or tense your shoulders. It might help to do this in front of a mirror, so you can be sure that your shoulders remain level. Try to hold this position for a minute – it is not as easy as it looks.

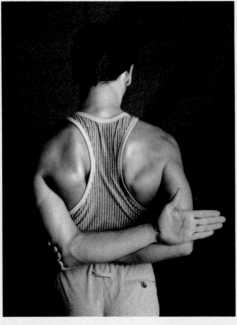

Half-nelson
Bring your left arm behind your back, holding it at the elbow with your right arm and pulling it back and to the right, creating a stretch in your shoulder. Make sure both elbows remain bent and your body stays upright. Hold the stretch for around 30 seconds, then switch arms.

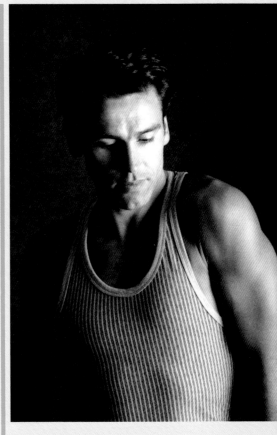

Shoulder rolls
Standing with your arms relaxed by your sides, raise one shoulder up to your ear, then rotate it slowly forward, then down, then draw it back and up again toward your ear, keeping the movement as full and circular as you can. Do this three times in one direction, then reverse for three times, before changing to the other side. Pay attention to keeping the rest of your body as still as possible without tensing, leaving all the movement to your shoulders.

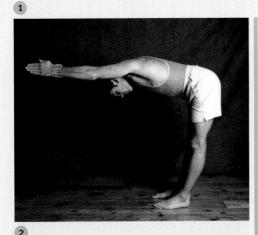

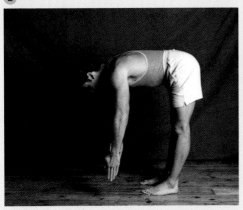

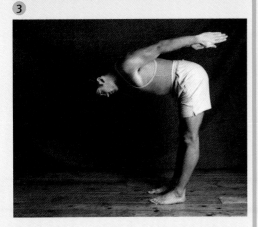

Chicken wings

This might remind you of the kind of playing around you did when you were a child. Make fists and place them in your armpits, then flap your arms vigorously up and down, resisting the temptation to cluck merrily. Flap away for around 30 seconds.

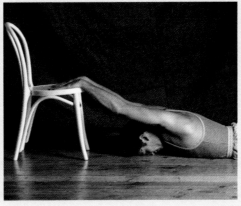

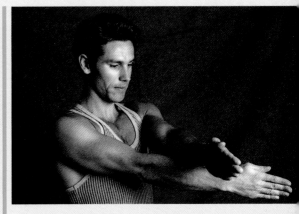

Scissors

Stand upright with your feet hips' width apart and extend your arms straight out in front of you, with your palms facing. Cross your arms, then recross them with vigorous but controlled movements, alternating which arm is on top. Move them up and down your body from shoulder level to hip level and back up again. Do this twice.

Pendulum

Standing with your feet hips' width apart, bend over from the waist until your upper body is roughly parallel to the floor, but you are not straining at all. If the position is uncomfortable, raise your body slightly. Swing your arms freely forward from the shoulders, aiming to get them over your head (1), and on the return (2) swing them until they are higher than your hips (3). Keep your body still, focusing the movement in your arms and shoulders. Repeat at least 10 times, enjoying the free and easy movement.

Shoulder hang

Lying face down on the floor and with about eight inches between your head and a chair, lift each arm and rest the palm of each hand on the seat of the chair. Straightening both arms, let your head drop down toward the floor. Try to relax there for up to a minute. Make sure you rest before you try it again.

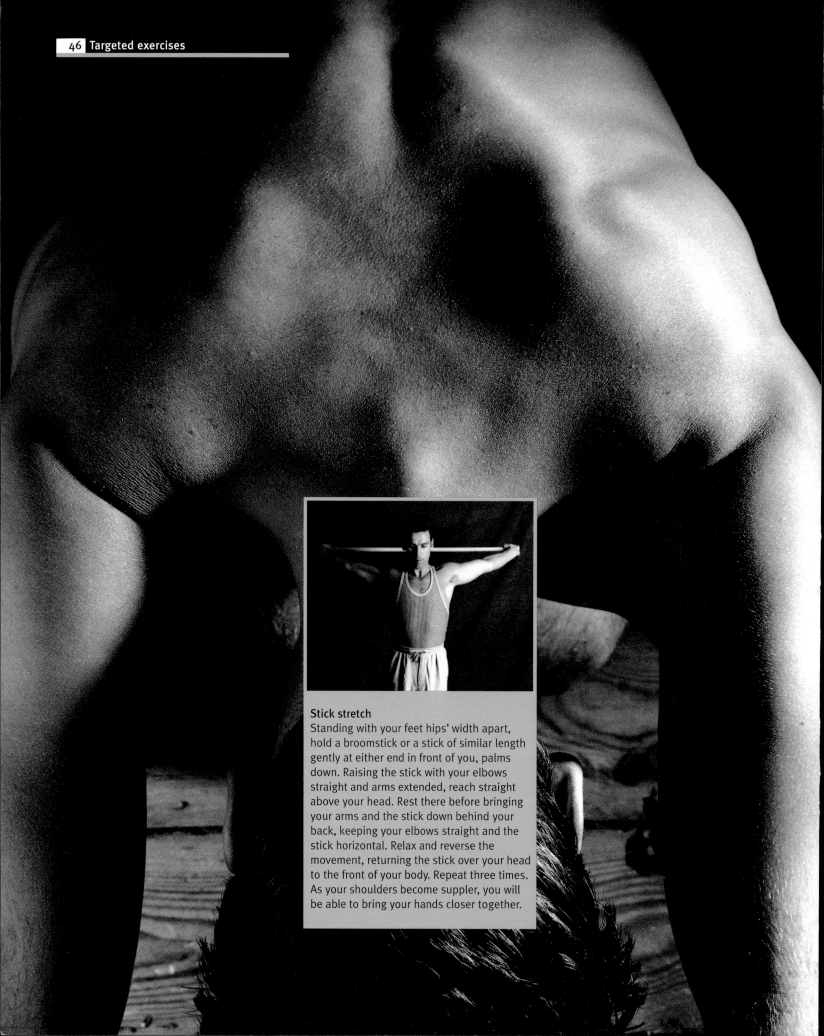

Stick stretch

Standing with your feet hips' width apart, hold a broomstick or a stick of similar length gently at either end in front of you, palms down. Raising the stick with your elbows straight and arms extended, reach straight above your head. Rest there before bringing your arms and the stick down behind your back, keeping your elbows straight and the stick horizontal. Relax and reverse the movement, returning the stick over your head to the front of your body. Repeat three times. As your shoulders become suppler, you will be able to bring your hands closer together.

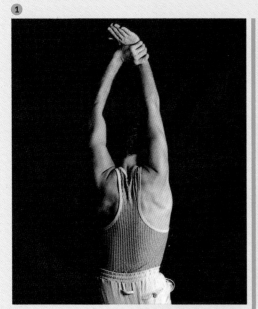

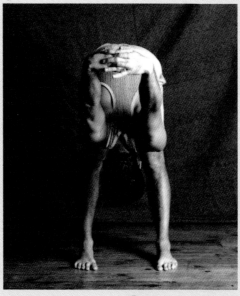

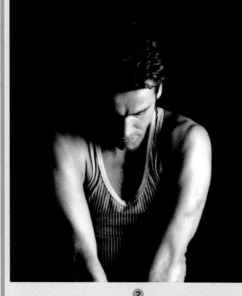

Cowface

Standing or sitting comfortably on the floor, raise your right arm above your head, perhaps using your left arm to tug it gently up a little higher, so that the right side of your body is stretched (1). Bend your right elbow so your forearm is lowered behind your head. Holding your right elbow with your left hand, nudge your right arm a little lower, increasing the stretch in your shoulder, but making sure your right elbow points upward. Bring your left arm around and clasp hands (2), or if you cannot quite reach hold onto your shirt. Hold for around 30 seconds, or as long as it is comfortable. If this is very difficult, simply repeat the first stage without trying to clasp hands. Switch arms and repeat.

Clasped hand forward bend

Standing with your legs hips' width apart, clasp your hands behind your back, interlacing your fingers with your palms facing up. Bend forward from the waist, letting your arms follow naturally (1). You should feel a stretch along the back of your body and especially in your shoulders. Then release your hands and let your arms dangle freely (2). Nod your head gently in little yes's and no's, feeling a release in your neck.

Shoulder fold

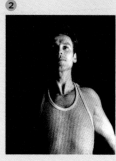

Sitting on a chair or standing comfortably with your arms by your sides, draw both of your shoulders forward, keeping them low and level, as if they would meet in front of your body (1). Hold this position for 10 seconds. Then reverse the stretch, pulling your shoulders backward as if they would meet behind your back (2). Again, hold the stretch for 10 seconds.

Arms and hands
targeted exercises

Think about the minute but complex actions needed to tie your shoelaces or write a note. Compare this to the burden of carrying shopping and you begin to get a picture of the varied daily workload endured by your hands and arms. Many recreational activities are also tough on them – think of the effort needed for tennis or even for knitting or embroidery. Our hands and arms rarely get a chance to relax.

It is no wonder that this area of the body often harbors stiffness and discomfort. Gentle stretching and manipulation will encourage flexibility and strength, and help to relieve the pressure on these often neglected parts of the body.

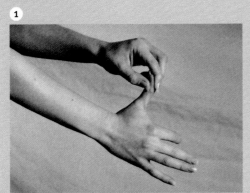

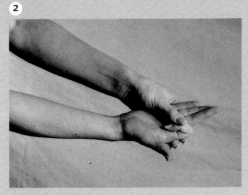

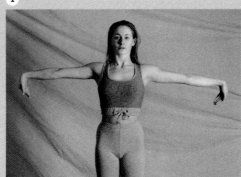

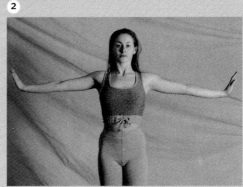

Thumb and finger rotations
This isn't so much an exercise but rather a gentle massage of the hands that is both pleasant and beneficial. Beginning with the thumb, hold each finger in turn lightly with the other hand and gently rotate it to its limit in both directions (1). Then, starting again with the thumb, gently press the fingers and thumb as far down toward your arm as possible, then as far into the palm of the hand (2). Complete one hand, then move to the other.

"T" shape with wrist action
Standing comfortably, slowly raise your arms out sideways, keeping them straight at the elbows, until they are horizontal to the floor. Extend them fully, stretching your fingers out, at the same time making sure you do not raise or tense your shoulders. Flex your wrists up and down 30 times (1 and 2), then lower your arms and shake them gently to relax. Raise them again, and this time rotate your hands 15 times in one direction and 15 times in the other.

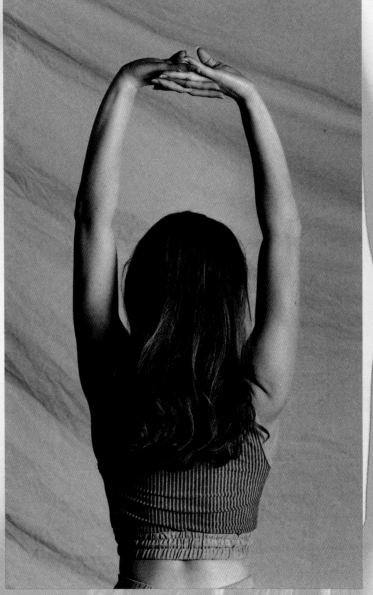

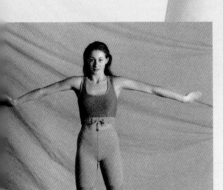

Wing flap
Stand comfortably with your feet hips' width apart and your arms by your sides. Turn your arms so your palms face outward with the thumbs to the rear. Slowly raise your arms as high as they can go, without hunching your shoulders, then lower them equally slowly. Repeat this five times.

Palm rotations
Extend your left arm straight in front of you with the palm facing up. Rotate the palm outward (clockwise) from the shoulder, using your right hand to increase the rotation when required. Hold for 15 seconds and repeat on the other side, rotating the right palm outward (counterclockwise).

Tower
Sitting on a chair with your feet flat on the floor, interlock your fingers and, with your palms facing up, stretch your arms above your head. Make sure your elbows are straight and your upper arms are pulled behind your ears. Relax and breathe. Hold for about a minute before resting and then repeating. Release your fingers and clasp again with the other thumb on top before repeating twice more.

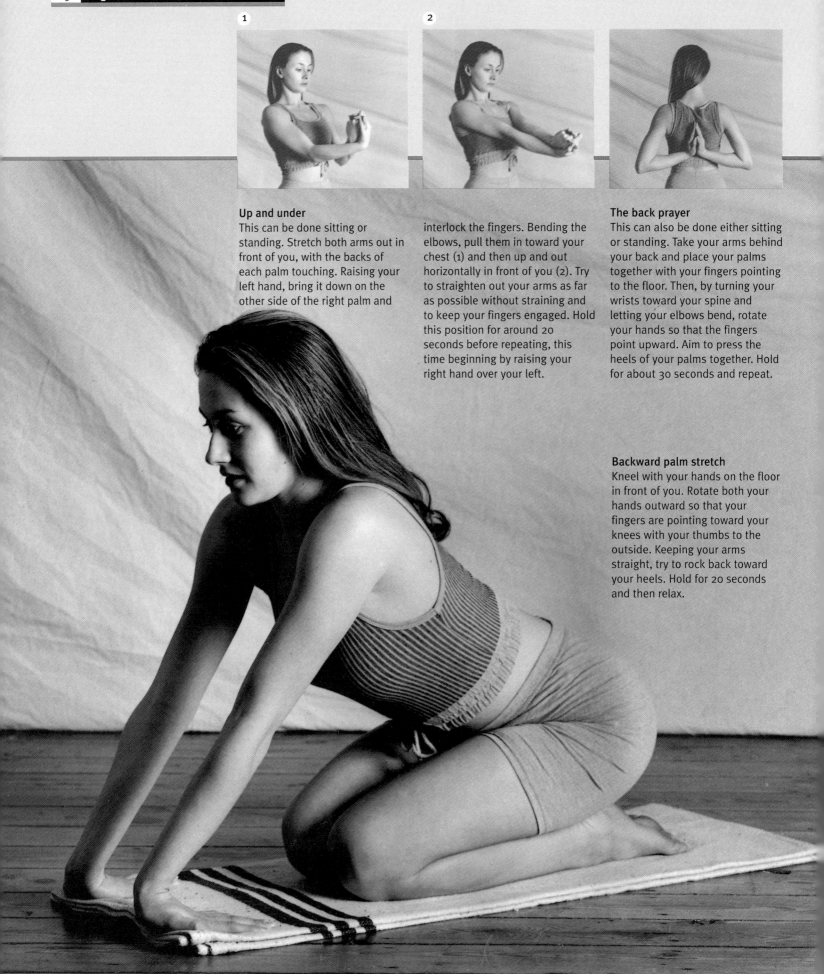

Up and under

This can be done sitting or standing. Stretch both arms out in front of you, with the backs of each palm touching. Raising your left hand, bring it down on the other side of the right palm and interlock the fingers. Bending the elbows, pull them in toward your chest (1) and then up and out horizontally in front of you (2). Try to straighten out your arms as far as possible without straining and to keep your fingers engaged. Hold this position for around 20 seconds before repeating, this time beginning by raising your right hand over your left.

The back prayer

This can also be done either sitting or standing. Take your arms behind your back and place your palms together with your fingers pointing to the floor. Then, by turning your wrists toward your spine and letting your elbows bend, rotate your hands so that the fingers point upward. Aim to press the heels of your palms together. Hold for about 30 seconds and repeat.

Backward palm stretch

Kneel with your hands on the floor in front of you. Rotate both your hands outward so that your fingers are pointing toward your knees with your thumbs to the outside. Keeping your arms straight, try to rock back toward your heels. Hold for 20 seconds and then relax.

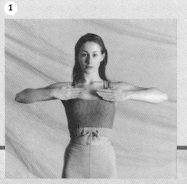
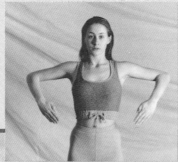
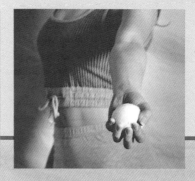

Traffic cop

Standing comfortably upright, extend your arms straight out sideways, keeping them level with your shoulders and parallel to the floor. Turn your palms backward and swing your lower arms from the elbow, bringing them in toward your chest until they are level with your shoulders (1), then return them to the starting position (2). Repeat 20 times, keeping your arms parallel to your shoulders throughout.

Tennis ball squeeze

This is exactly what it sounds like. Take a tennis ball in each hand and squeeze repeatedly as hard as you can without straining. You can vary this by raising or lowering your arms, or bringing them in front of your body. Just keep your elbows straight but not locked while you are squeezing. You can do this as often as you like and for as long as you like.

Penguin flap

This is very similar to the wing flap on page 49. Standing comfortably upright, bring your arms behind your back, keeping your elbows straight and your palms facing up. Holding the rest of your body still, raise your arms as high as you comfortably can behind you, then lower them. Repeat this 10 times, feeling the stretch toward the outsides of your arms.

Back targeted exercises

Your spine is designed to bend in four directions: forward, backward, sideways, and rotationally or twisting. But in the normal course of things, we bend over forward most often, and hold tense, unnatural forward positions. Think of leaning over to write, to eat, to wash dishes, to read the paper, to make the bed. The result of this imbalance, for many people, is back pain.

These exercises are designed to restore a natural range of movement to the back. They will also help to strengthen your back and its supporting muscles. The benefits will soon be apparent, from more enhanced and attractive posture to freer breathing. With any exercises involving the back, however, it is vital to work very gently and carefully, aiming for gradual and consistent improvement.

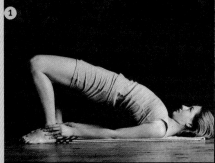

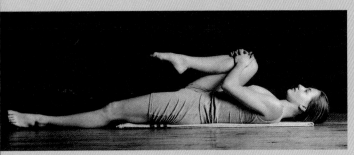

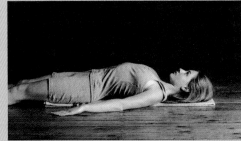

Knee to chest stretch
Lying on your back on the floor, bend your right knee and, clasping it with your hands, pull your knee toward your chest, bouncing it gently. After about 30 seconds, relax and repeat the exercise on the other leg. For a slightly more challenging version of this exercise, you can try the head to knee stretch below.

Small bridge stretch
Lying on the floor on your back with your legs stretched straight out and your hands resting lightly on your hip bones or the floor, simply flatten your back until it is all touching the floor, then arch it so that only your shoulders and buttocks touch the floor. Repeat 10 times.

Bridge pose
This advanced exercise should be taken in stages to begin with. Lie on your back on the floor with your knees bent and your feet hips' width apart. Hold your ankles – if you can't reach, place your palms flat on the floor with your arms extended. Lift your pelvis, trying to raise it as high as possible (1). Hold for 15 seconds then come down slowly, one vertebra at a time, starting from the top of your spine.

Repeat this exercise, but this time place your hands palms down under your shoulders with your fingers pointing toward your feet. Straighten your elbows and lift your pelvis and abdomen into the air. Rest for a few moments on your head. To take the stretch even further, you can straighten your elbows and knees as much as possible, arching your back (2). After about 15 seconds lower yourself gently, one vertebra at a time.

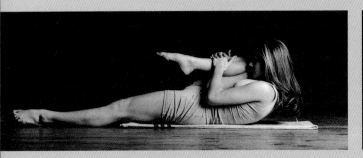

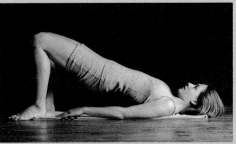

Head to knee stretch
This is a slightly more difficult version of the knee to chest stretch above. As before, begin by lying on the floor and, clasping your right knee with your hands, pull the knee toward your chest. This time, however, lift your head and try to touch your knee with your forehead. As an enhancement to this stretch, you might like to try touching your knee with your nose or your ear. After about 30 seconds, relax and repeat on the other side.

Pelvic thrust
Lie on your back on the floor with your knees bent and your feet hips' width apart. Keeping your feet and shoulders still, raise your pelvis into the air as high as it will go, then lower it slowly. Repeat 10 times. When you lower yourself for the last time, do so very slowly, placing one vertebra on the floor at a time, beginning at the top of your spine.

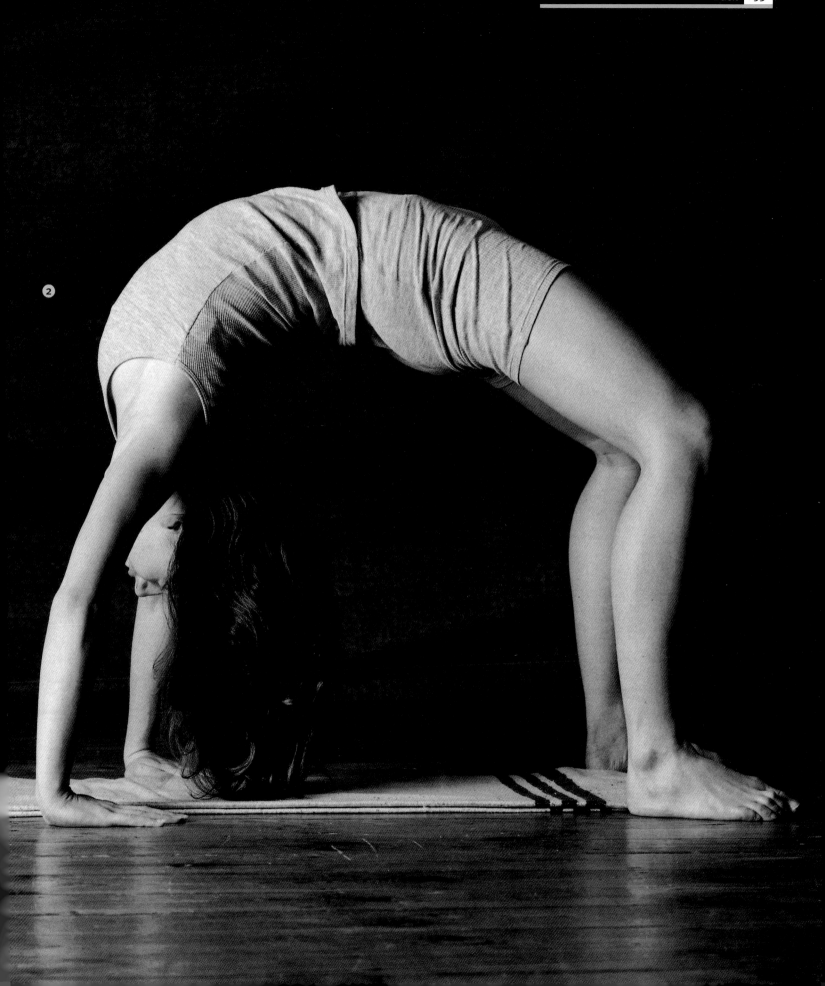

Sitting spinal twist

The description of this stretch makes it sound complicated, but it really isn't difficult at all. Sit on the floor with both legs straight out in front of you and your spine upright. Pick up your right leg and, bending the knee, put your foot down on the left side of your left knee. Put your right hand on the floor behind your right buttock, keeping your elbow straight. Lift your left arm and, keeping the elbow straight, bring it over your upright right knee and place your left hand lightly on your right leg. Turn to look as far as you can over your right shoulder, thinking of raising your lower back. Hold for a minute or as long as it is comfortable. Just before you release, turn to look in front of you. Relax and switch sides. To get into the position from now on, remember "opposite arm to leg" – the arm that goes over is the opposite one to the upright leg.

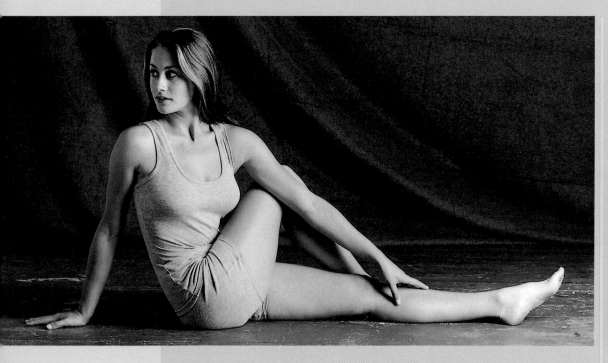

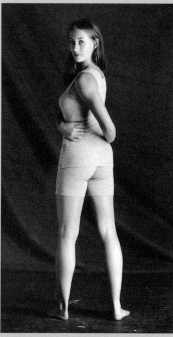

Standing twist

Stand firmly with your feet hips' width apart. Keeping your thighs and knees facing forward, twist your pelvis and upper body so you are looking behind yourself. Reaching around with your arms, try to twist a little further with every breath, always keeping your shoulders level. After 30 seconds, reverse the twist.

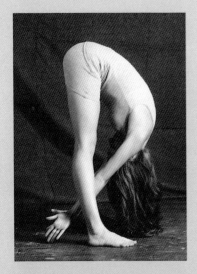

Forward bend and hang

With your feet hips' width apart and knees loose, tip over from the waist and reach to your feet. The upper body should feel as if it is hanging from your hips. Keeping your weight spread across your feet, relax your stomach with each breath and let your back get looser. When you've had enough, slowly roll up. Think of your back getting straighter one vertebra at a time.

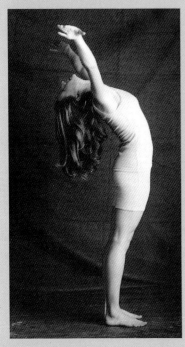

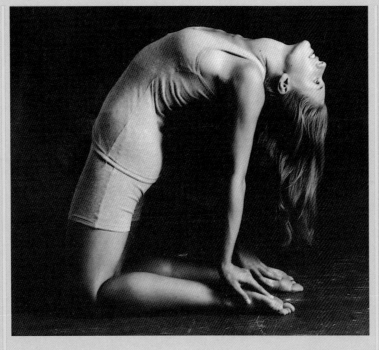

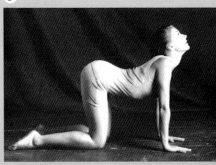

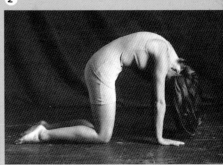

Backward bend

Separate your feet a little wider than your hips for better balance, and place your hands on your hips. Tightening your buttocks, stretch backward with your hands running down the back of your thighs for balance. You should feel the stretch both in your upper back and in your abdominal muscles. When you are confident in your balance and your back is more supple, you can do the backward bend with your hands raised over your head.

Camel stretch

This is an advanced backward bending stretch. Kneeling up on the floor with your legs a little wider than hips' width apart, gently reach back and place your right hand on top of your right foot, keeping your pelvis up and facing forward. When you are comfortable and balanced, carefully lower your left hand so it is on top of your left foot, and drop your head back. Keep your buttocks squeezed together so your lower back is not strained. For a stronger stretch, push forward with your hips.

Cat arching

Kneeling with your hands on the floor directly under your shoulders, curve your back downward to hollow it, at the same time raising your head up (1). Then arch your back upward to hunch it and drop your head (2). Do this about 10 times.

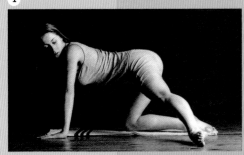

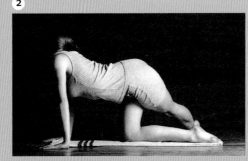

Footsie

Resting on your hands and knees, stretch your left leg out sideways, keeping it straight, with your toes resting on the floor. Turn your head to the left to look at your foot (1). Now swing your leg around behind you, keeping it straight and close to the ground, and turn your head to the right until you see it again (2). Return it to the starting point, and repeat twice more before changing to the other leg.

Sideways leg raising

This is a physiotherapy exercise. Lie on your left side on the floor. Rest your head on your left hand and place your right hand in front of you for support. Making sure that your body is straight, lock your right knee and flex your feet, then lift your right leg up as far as it will go. Slowly lower the leg and repeat 10 times. Relax and repeat on the other side.

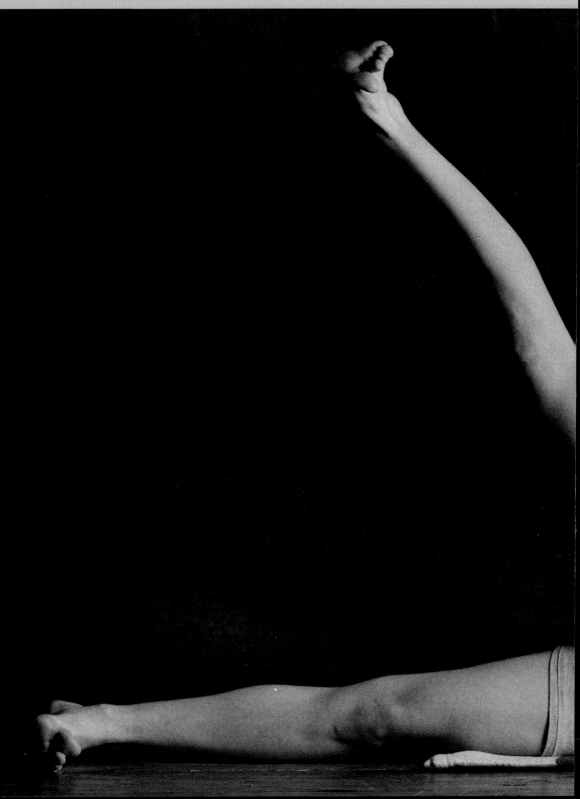

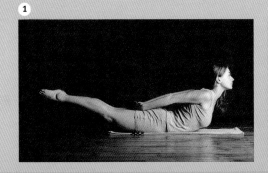

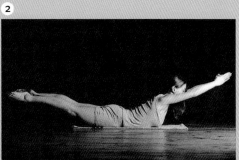

The boat pose and variations

Lying on the floor on your stomach, clasp your hands behind your back and straighten your elbows. Breathing in, raise your head, upper body, and legs, and hold for as long as is comfortable (1).To vary this, keep your arms extended straight out in front of you (2). Once you have raised your upper body and legs in this position, you can rock back and forth vigorously, like a boat tossed on the waves.

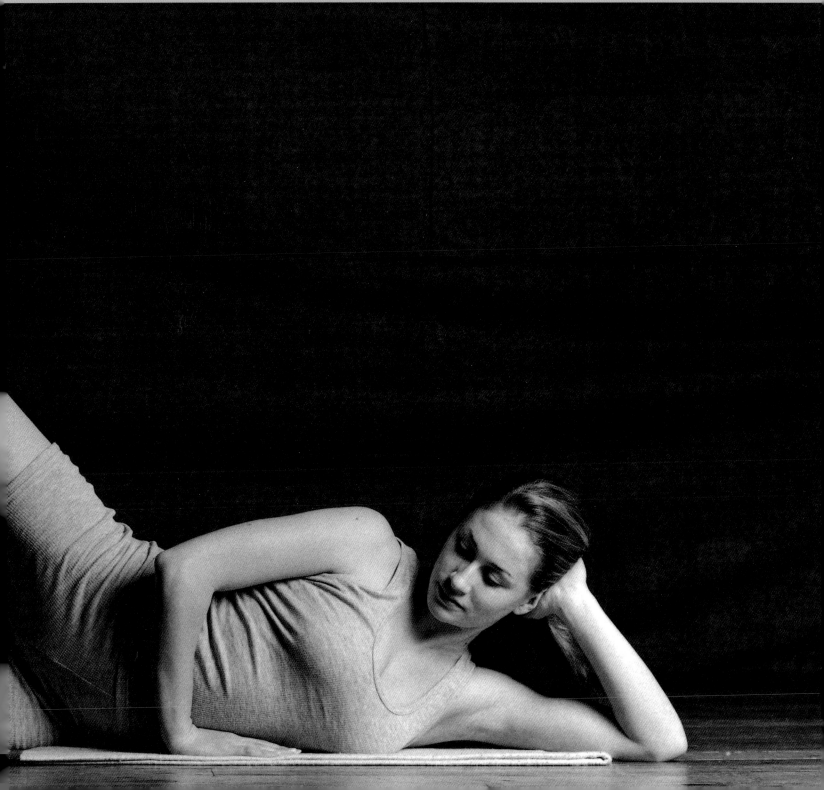

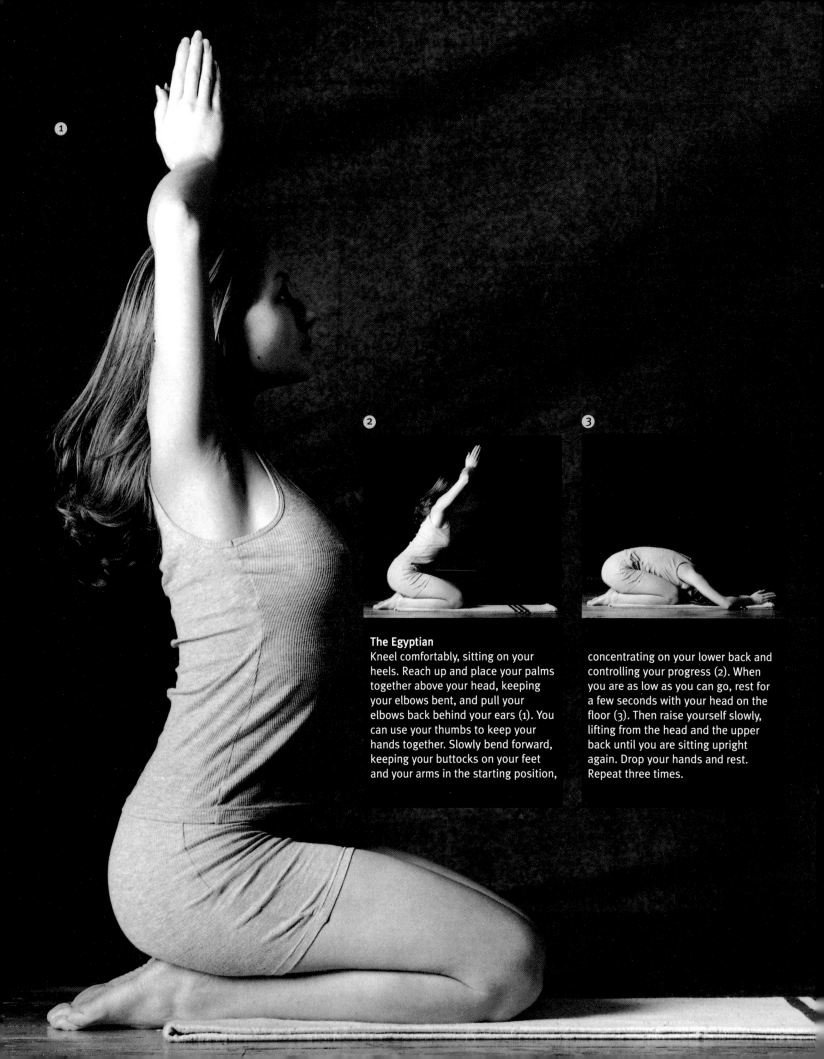

The Egyptian

Kneel comfortably, sitting on your heels. Reach up and place your palms together above your head, keeping your elbows bent, and pull your elbows back behind your ears (1). You can use your thumbs to keep your hands together. Slowly bend forward, keeping your buttocks on your feet and your arms in the starting position, concentrating on your lower back and controlling your progress (2). When you are as low as you can go, rest for a few seconds with your head on the floor (3). Then raise yourself slowly, lifting from the head and the upper back until you are sitting upright again. Drop your hands and rest. Repeat three times.

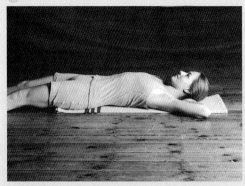

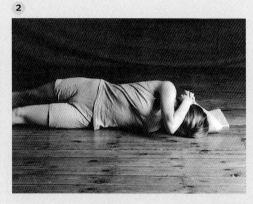

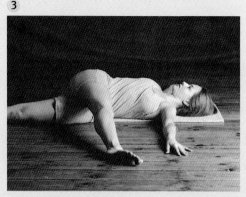

Lying spinal twist

These are two kinds of twists that you can do lying flat on your back, even in bed. One concentrates on the upper spine and the other on the lower spine. For the upper spine, clasp your hands behind your head, letting your elbows flop flat on the floor (1). Keeping your heels on the floor, turn your upper body to the left, trying to touch your right elbow to the floor next to your left elbow (2). Hold for about 30 seconds then relax before turning the other way. For the lower spine, raise your right leg up and over your body, lowering it to the ground on your left side, keeping your shoulders flat on the floor (3). You can heighten the stretch by turning your head to the right.

The plough

This is a very powerful yoga stretch for your whole body. Lie on your back on the floor with your arms by your sides and your palms down. Make sure there are several feet of clear space above your head. Bending your knees, raise your legs to your chest then swing them over your head until your feet touch the floor and you are resting on your neck.

If your feet do not touch the floor, position a chair or a stool to rest them on. Keeping your chin toward your chest, clasp your hands with your arms extended and aim to rest your toes on the floor. You will find that pulling your elbows closer together will enhance the stretch. If you find that your breathing is restricted, do not worry – it will become easier as you relax.

To enhance the stretch further, release your arms and bend your knees, letting them rest next to your ears. Reach up and hold your feet (2). When you are ready to come down, keep your legs bent and close to your chest and let your arms support your back as you roll down slowly, one vertebra at a time.

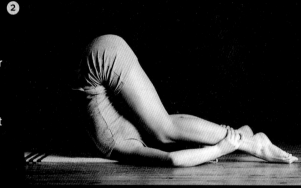

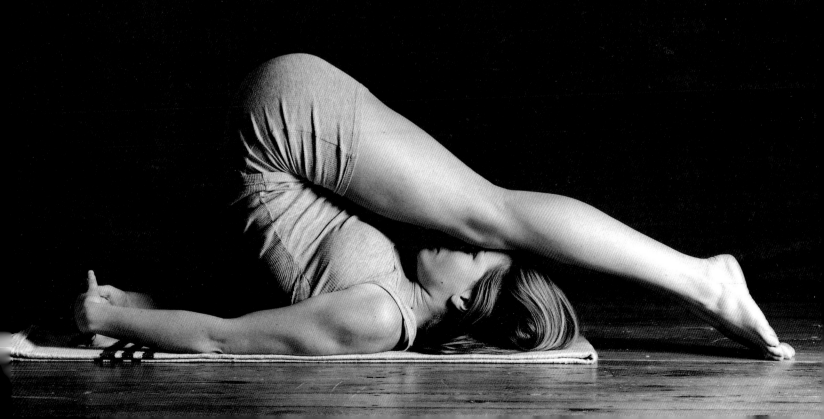

Pointer
This is a stretch and a balance all in one. Beginning on your hands and knees looking straight ahead, lift and extend your right leg while keeping your hips level and pointing your toes. When you are balanced, raise and extend your left arm. Hold this position for 10 seconds, then relax and repeat on the other side.

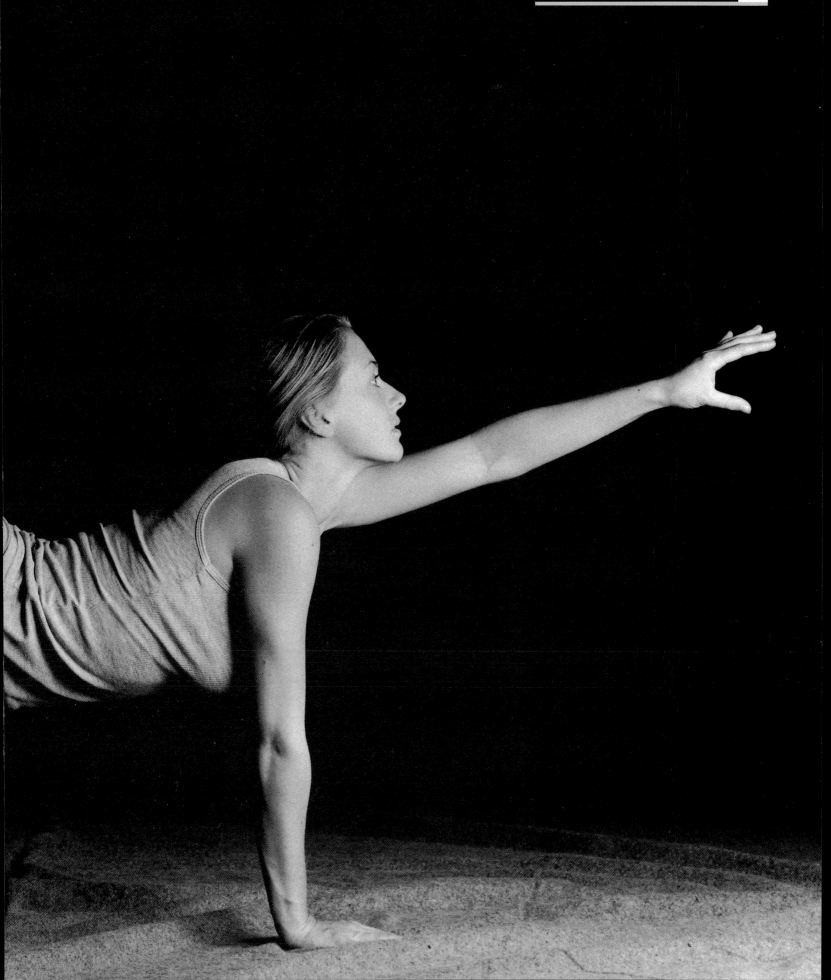

Ironing board back

Begin by standing upright with your arms raised straight above your head and your palms together. Keeping your ears between your arms and your back straight, bend at the waist until your upper body is parallel to the floor. Aim to stay in this position, with your back straight, for 30 seconds. If this is very difficult, you can begin practicing by holding onto a window sill or the back of a chair for support.

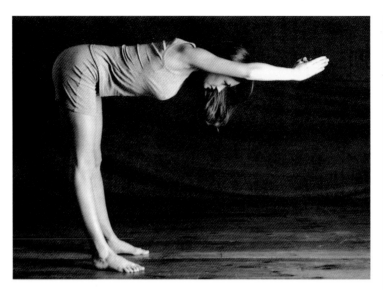

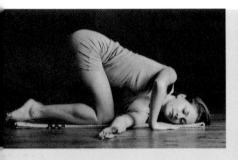

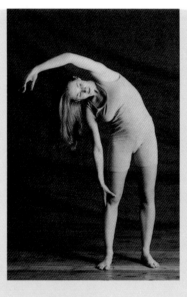

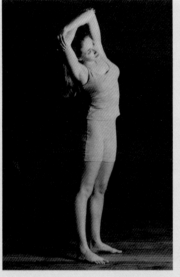

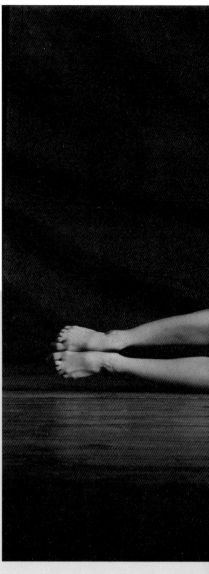

Kneeling twist

Begin on your hands and knees on the floor. Pick up your left hand and, turning it palm up, slide it as far as you can along the floor between your right arm and your right leg, twisting your left shoulder and bending your right arm, until you are resting on the left side of your head and the top of your left shoulder. Hold for 10 seconds and repeat twice before reversing the exercise.

Elbow clasp side bend

Standing, or sitting upright and relaxed on a chair with your feet flat on the floor, raise both arms above your head and clasp each elbow in the opposite hand. Pull your upper arms as far behind your ears as possible. Keeping the elbows high and back, bend your upper body slowly to the right. Relax and breathe. Hold for about 10 seconds and then repeat on the other side. Aim to stretch at least three times on each side.

Crescent stretch

Keeping your feet flat and hips' width apart, raise your left arm and bend slowly over to your right, without bending either forward or backward at the waist. You should feel a strong stretch all along your side. When you are comfortable, turn your head up slightly. Hold this for 10 seconds then switch to the other side. Do this twice on each side.

Sideways body raising

Lie on your left side with your left arm straight out in line with your body, the palm flat on the floor and your left ear resting on your left arm. For balance, your right arm should be in front of you, palm flat on the floor. Using this arm as support, slowly raise your head and upper body as high as you can, keeping your legs together on the floor and not twisting your trunk. When you are as high as you can go, slowly lower yourself to the start position. Do this five times.

Once you become confident, try raising your legs off the floor as you raise your body (see above).

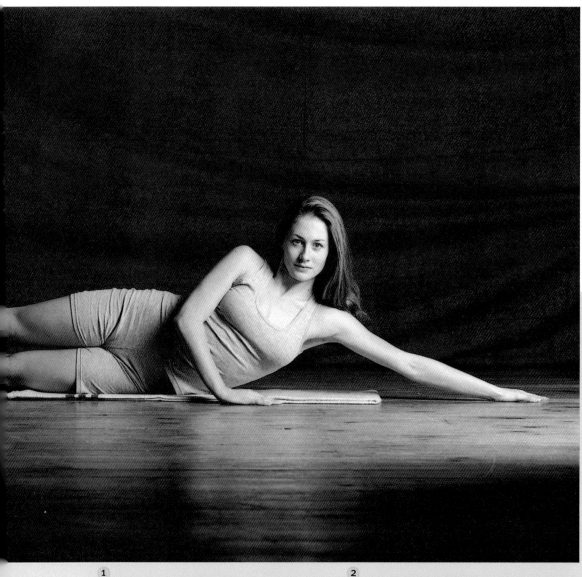

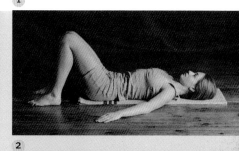

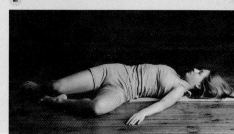

"J" twist

Lying on your back on the floor with your knees bent and together, place your feet flat on the floor about a foot apart (1). Keeping your shoulders flat on the ground, drop your knees toward the floor to the left. Your ultimate aim is to touch your left foot to your right knee without strain (2). If this is easy, gently work your legs, keeping them touching, so that you draw your right foot up toward your back, making a "J" shape with your body. Hold for 20 seconds and repeat on the other side.

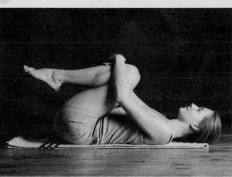

Cradle

Lying on your back on the floor, lift both your knees and, clasping them with your hands, pull them toward your chest (1). Relax and gently rock from side to side, turning your head in the opposite direction from your legs (2): that is, as your legs move to the right, your head moves to the left, and vice versa. Continue to rock gently for about 45 seconds.

Cobra with variations

Lying on the floor on your stomach, place your hands flat on the floor with your elbows bent and thumbs level with your armpits. Raise your head up slowly, arching your back. Do not use your arms to push – rather let your back and your abdomen do the work. Hold this for 10 seconds then try to raise a bit higher for 10 seconds.

On the opposite page there are a number of enhancements to this basic pose, which you can add as you become stronger and more flexible. Always begin with the basic stretch and listen to your body, checking whether you are ready to take it further. Some days it might better to keep it simple.

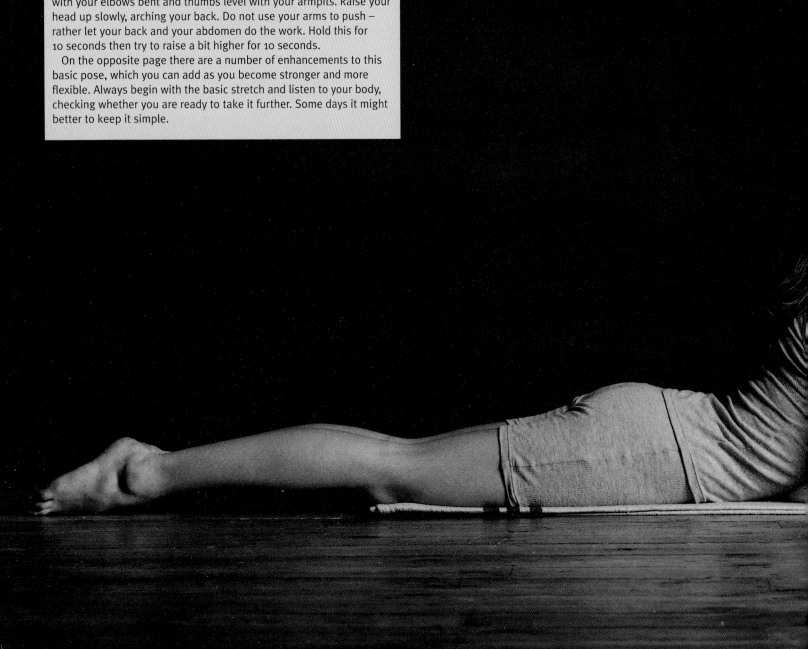

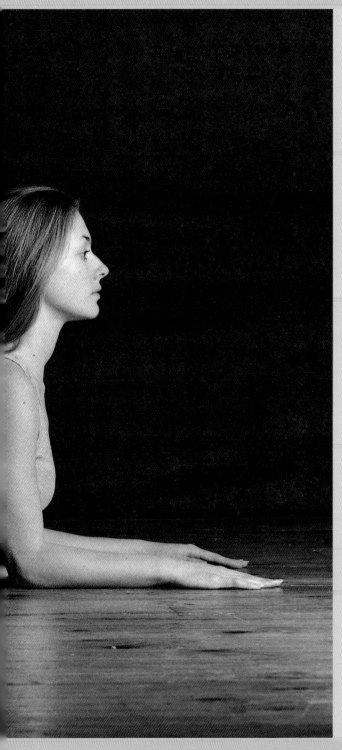

1

From the basic cobra position:

lift your hands a few inches from the floor without letting your body drop (1). Hold this for 10 seconds.

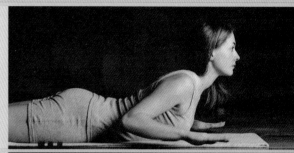

2

turn to the right, trying to see the back of your body and even your left foot (2). Face forward again, then turn to the left.

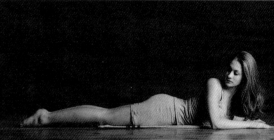

3

straighten your arms, tuck your toes under and lift your body an inch or two off the floor (3). Hold for a few seconds then relax.

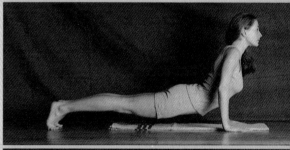

4

straighten your arms, tuck your toes under, and lift your body an inch or two off the floor. Raise your left leg and cross it over your right leg. Turn your head to look over your right shoulder (4). Hold this for a few seconds then reverse.

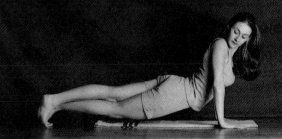

5

straighten your arms, tuck your toes under and lift your body an inch or two off the floor. Raise and lower first your right leg (5) then your left leg.

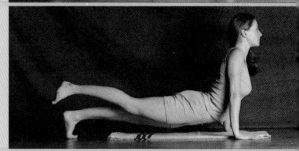

Stomach
targeted exercises

A flat tummy is an essential part of looking and feeling thin and healthy. We all want the abdominal muscles of a Greek god or supermodel, and this does not need to be an impossible dream. Keep this in mind if at first some of the exercises in this section seem difficult.

On a purely practical level, a strong abdomen protects your lower back from having to take unnecessary strain, because weak stomach muscles mean that your back has to take on extra work. A few minutes a day and you will find that your posture will improve, you will look and feel better, and you might save yourself back trouble in the future. At the very least, you are bound to find it easier to fasten the top button of your jeans.

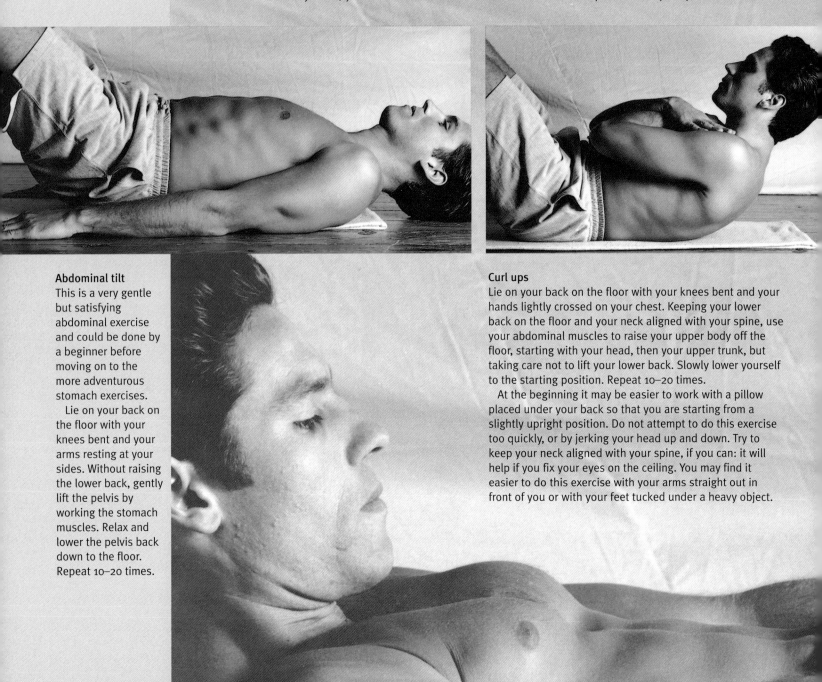

Abdominal tilt
This is a very gentle but satisfying abdominal exercise and could be done by a beginner before moving on to the more adventurous stomach exercises.

Lie on your back on the floor with your knees bent and your arms resting at your sides. Without raising the lower back, gently lift the pelvis by working the stomach muscles. Relax and lower the pelvis back down to the floor. Repeat 10–20 times.

Curl ups
Lie on your back on the floor with your knees bent and your hands lightly crossed on your chest. Keeping your lower back on the floor and your neck aligned with your spine, use your abdominal muscles to raise your upper body off the floor, starting with your head, then your upper trunk, but taking care not to lift your lower back. Slowly lower yourself to the starting position. Repeat 10–20 times.

At the beginning it may be easier to work with a pillow placed under your back so that you are starting from a slightly upright position. Do not attempt to do this exercise too quickly, or by jerking your head up and down. Try to keep your neck aligned with your spine, if you can: it will help if you fix your eyes on the ceiling. You may find it easier to do this exercise with your arms straight out in front of you or with your feet tucked under a heavy object.

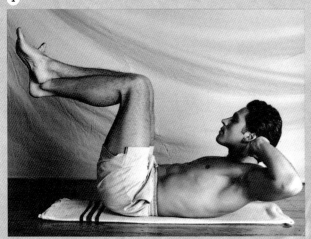

Crunchies

The following exercises are more advanced and you may wish to wait a little before attempting them. Always remember to keep your lower back on the floor. Try to keep your neck in line with your spine.

Lie on the floor with your fingers gently touching behind your ears. Lift your legs and cross your ankles, bending your knees at 90 degrees. Then, without jerking, lift your head toward your knees until you feel a pull in your stomach (1). Relax back down and repeat 10–20 times, recrossing your ankles in the other direction halfway through.

As a variation, you can pull your knees toward your chest as you lift your head, returning your legs to the starting position as you drop your head back to the floor. Alternatively, you can keep both legs straight up in the air as you do your crunchies(2).

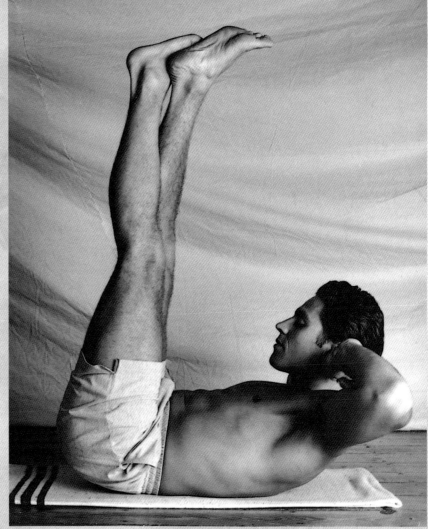

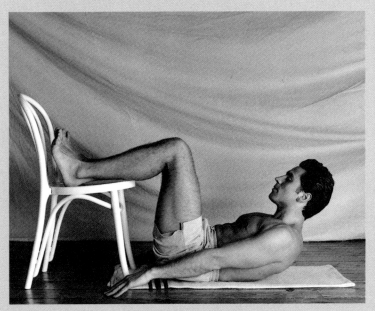

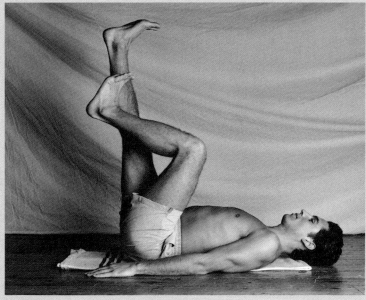

Almost sitting

This is a good way to prepare for more some of the more rigorous stomach exercises, strengthening you and warming you up. Lying on your back on the floor, place your calves on the seat of a chair and keep your arms relaxed by your side. Gently lift your head and shoulders, raising your upper body toward your legs, then lower yourself gently back down to the floor. Repeat 10 times. If this is difficult, place a cushion under your head and shoulders at the beginning to give your body a head start.

Air cycling

Lying on the floor on your back with your arms by your sides and palms flat on the floor, raise your legs straight up in the air and move them as if you were pedaling a bicycle. Vary the speed from time to time, sometimes pedaling furiously and at other times taking a more leisurely pace. Keep going for around two minutes. If you would like to work harder, you can do so by lifting your lower back off the floor and supporting it with your hands as you pedal.

Zombie

Lie on the floor on your back. Place your palms on your thighs and slowly roll up through your back, sliding your arms down your legs as you do, until you can touch your toes. Relax there before reversing the process, rolling down slowly, one vertebra at a time, as your hands slide back up. Make sure your hands remain relaxed along your legs throughout.

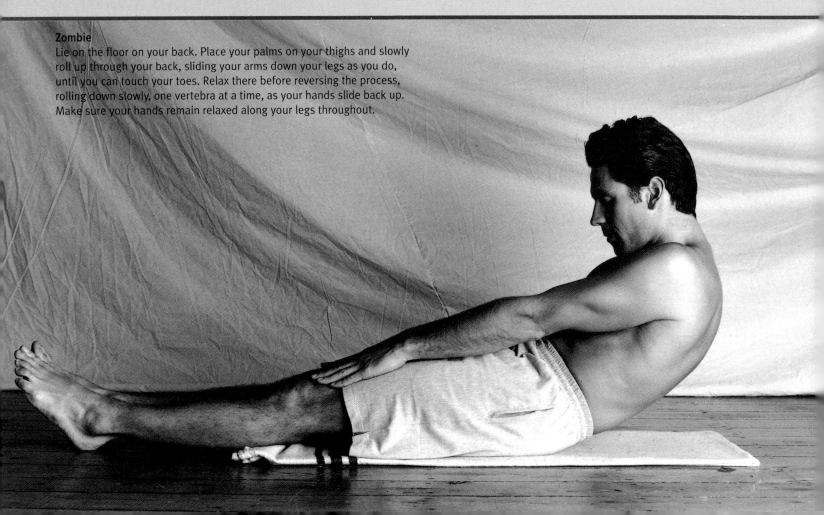

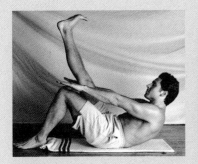

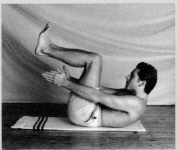

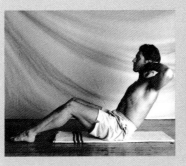

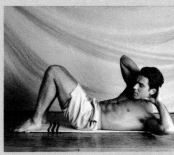

"V" kick

Begin by lying on the floor on your back with your arms extended behind your head, your right leg straight out in front of you, and your left knee bent and pointing to the ceiling. As you breathe out, sit up, keeping your back straight and bringing your arms over your head at the same time as you lift your right leg, keeping it straight and drawing it between your arms toward your chest. Return to the starting position, take a deep breath and repeat this five times, synchronizing your breathing with the movement, then switch legs.

Leg claps

Begin by lying flat on the floor on your back with your arms by your sides. Breathe in and, keeping your back straight, in one controlled movement sit up and raise your legs off the floor with knees bent. Bring your hands together under your bent knees to clap, then return to the floor. Repeat this movement as many times as you can without straining, aiming to do it 10 times.

Body lowering

This is the opposite to leg lowering (see below) – your legs stay still and your torso and head return to the floor. Sit on the floor with your knees slightly bent, pointing up to the ceiling, and clasp your hands behind your neck. Slowly lower your upper body to the floor for a count of 10, keeping your back straight. Resist the temptation to go too fast at the beginning, because you will only have to slow down later on – eventually you should try to increase the time it takes you to lower your body, working up to 15 and even 20 seconds.

Oblique curl

Lie on your back on the floor with your knees bent and hips' width apart and your fingertips resting lightly behind your ears. Keeping your lower back on the floor and your head in line with your spine, try to touch your left knee with your right elbow. Relax back to the floor and then try and touch your left knee with your right elbow. Relax back down to the starting position and repeat 10–20 times.

Leg lowering

Lie on your back on the floor with your legs straight up in the air. Try to hold for 30 seconds. If you want to do a little more work, walk a little in the air.

When you feel confident and strong you can try lowering your legs. Keeping your upper arms at your sides, interlace your fingers and rest your hands over your stomach. This will allow you to press down on your tummy and help you to keep your lower back on the floor as you continue the exercise. Flex your feet and very slowly lower your legs to the floor, keeping the legs straight. Repeat 10 times. For an enhancement to this exercise, do 10 repetitions without actually allowing the feet to touch the floor, instead letting them hover an inch above the ground before repeating.

It is very important that you take your time with this exercise – the slower you lower your legs, the greater the reward.

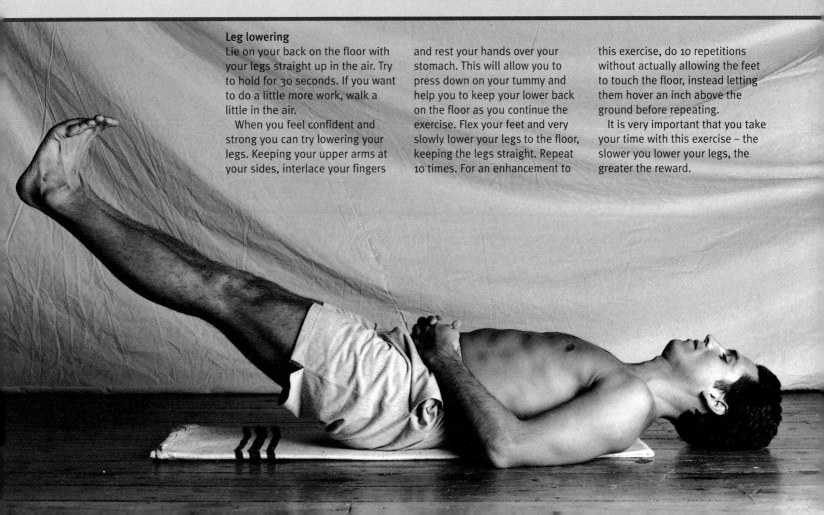

Hips and buttocks
targeted exercises

You might think that because the hips and buttocks are responsible for standing and walking, the two most common forms of exercise for all of us, this area of the body would be stronger and more flexible than the rest. But this is not the case.

To start with, walking is becoming almost the exception rather than the rule in our modern lifestyles. When we do walk, we limit the movement of our hips to backward and forward swings. But the hip is made up of a ball and socket joint, which means that it is capable of a wide range of movement in all directions. You only have to watch children playing in a park to see the full range of possible movement – they run, crawl, and climb throughout their games. However, there are natural inbuilt controls to the hips' range of movement, which is most limited in extending backward and freest in extending forward, for the sake of stability when standing. Loss of flexibility in the hip joint can cause discomfort as well as difficulty in walking.

The following exercises will release and strengthen your hips and buttocks, and you should find that your stride will improve with your posture. And if all that is not reason enough to exercise your hips every day, keep in mind that regular exercise of the hips and buttocks will tone up an area of the body that is always a preoccupation for the dieter.

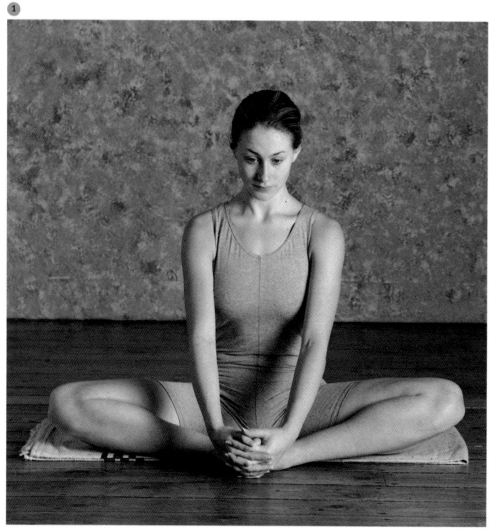

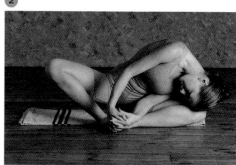

Butterfly
Sit on the floor with your knees bent and the soles of your feet touching. Hold your feet with your hands and pull them as close to your groin as you can without slouching in the lower back. The aim is to get your knees to touch the floor, so gently push down on your thighs with your elbows or lightly bounce your knees up and down. Hold the position (1) for between one and three minutes, and then relax.

You can add another dimension to this stretch by involving the rest of your body. Sitting in the butterfly position, turn from the waist and bend to touch your forehead to your left knee (2). Straighten and then bend to touch your forehead to your right knee.

Then, again from the waist, bend forward to touch your forehead to the floor in front of you without lifting your buttocks, stretching your arms out in front. You should aim to have a straight back, as if you were folding at the waist. Hold this position for as long as you find it comfortable.

Lying butterfly

This is as it sounds. Lie on your back on the floor with your knees bent and your heels touching. Drop your knees to push them as far apart as possible. To keep your lower back straight, you may want to tilt your pelvis upward slightly, which will push your back into the floor. Relax and hold the position for one to three minutes.

Baby sleeping pose

You may be more comfortable if you have a pillow under your knees for this one. Kneeling with your hands on the floor in front of you, spread your knees as wide as you can while keeping your big toes in contact. Shift your weight on to your hands and drop down onto your chest so that you are lying on your front.

You will find that your buttocks will stay in the air, and your feet will rise also. The stiffer the hips, the higher your buttocks. Try to relax in this position, letting your knees shift further apart as you do, and with luck your bottom will creep toward the floor. Hold for 30 seconds, return to your hands and knees, and repeat.

Diagonal knee-to-chest stretch

Lying comfortably on the floor on your back, bring your right knee up toward your chest. Holding your knee in your arms, draw it gently toward your left shoulder. Hold for 20 seconds, then release and switch to the other leg. Repeat five times on each leg.

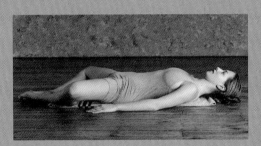

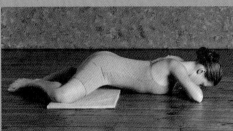

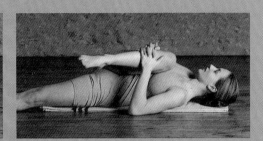

Hip lift

Sitting on the floor, bend your left knee, keeping your leg flat on the floor, and bring your foot in toward your groin. Then, supporting yourself with your left hand, bring your right leg behind you, bending your knee. Lift your right leg as high as you can without straining and lower it to the floor. Repeat this 20 times before switching over to the other side.

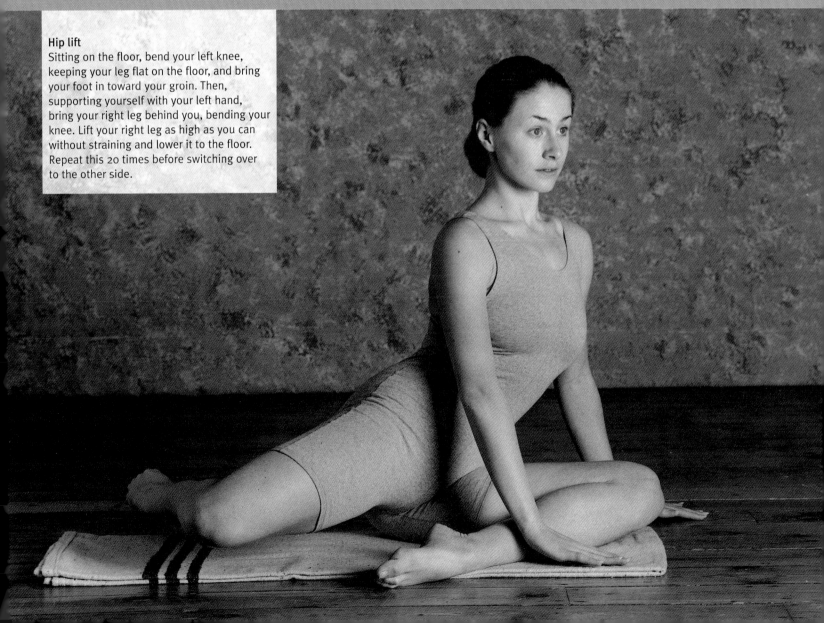

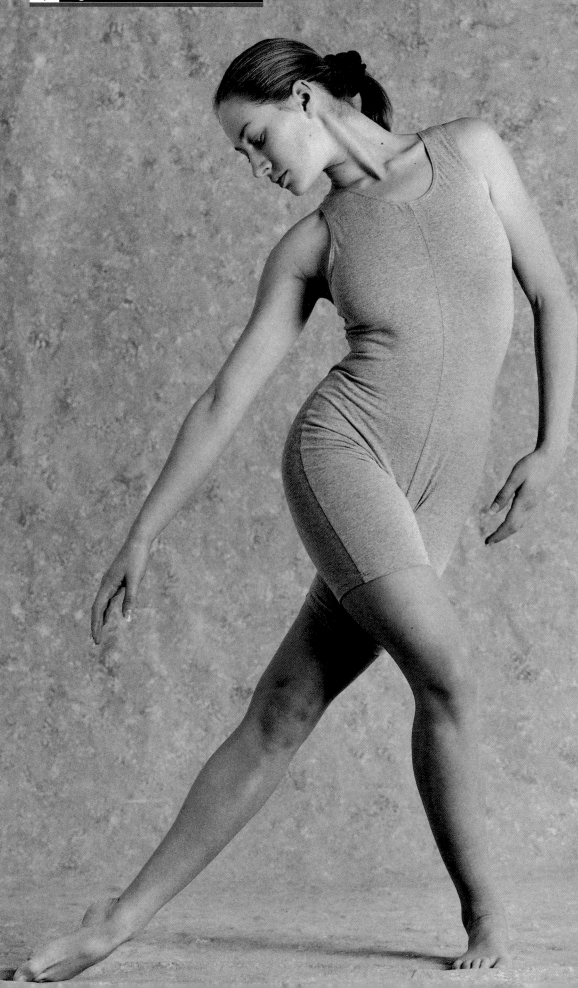

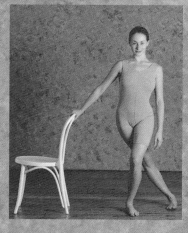

Cross-leg lean

Standing, place your right hand on the back of a chair or on a wall, keeping your arm straight. Bring your left leg in front of your right, keeping your feet in line. With your back straight and both feet flat on the floor, bend your left knee slightly and draw your right hip down and toward the chair. You should feel a pull up the outside of your right hip. Hold for five seconds then relax. Repeat three times, then change to the left side.

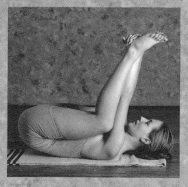

Frog's legs

Lying on your back on the floor, raise your knees up toward your chest. Widen your knees slightly so that they are more in line with your elbows and reach up and grab the insides of your feet. By now your legs should be bent from the knees at 90 degrees, and the soles of your feet should be facing the ceiling. Relax and hold the position for about 45 seconds before releasing and repeating.

Kneeling triangle
Kneeling upright on the floor, extend your left leg out at a right angle to your body. Without twisting your upper body, straighten your right arm and stretch it up and over your head toward your left foot. Meanwhile slide your left arm down your thigh toward your foot. Hold this position for about 15 seconds then repeat on the other side.

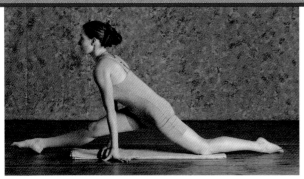

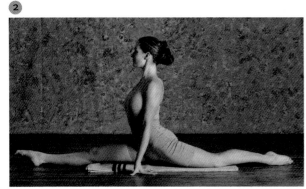

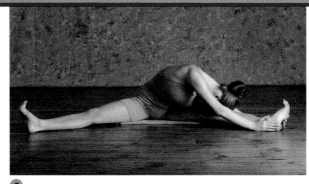

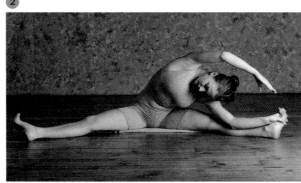

Full splits

It is possible, with the right kind of practice, to learn to do full splits, and the preparatory stretching is well worth it on its own. Begin by kneeling on the floor, with a cushion or a rolled-up towel under your knees to protect them if you want, placing your palms flat on the floor on either side of your hips for stability.

Stretch your right leg out in front of you until it can go no further, keeping it straight, and support your weight on your hands (1). Relax and hold for about 20 seconds, bearing some of your weight on your arms to avoid straining your legs, before lowering yourself gently to your right side (2). Relax and repeat on the left.

Sitting side splits with variations

Sit on the floor with your legs as wide as possible, making sure that your back is straight – if you find it very difficult to straighten your back, it is better to bring your legs in a little bit so that you are able to sit upright. Flex and point your feet 10 times. You can increase this stretch in a number of different ways.

Turn to face your left foot and bend down to reach it (1), keeping your back and shoulders level and aiming to rest your elbows on the floor on either side of your leg. Each time you breathe out, try to move a little deeper into the stretch. Raise yourself gently then repeat on the other side.

Facing forward, bend your body to the left, aiming to hold your left foot in your left hand with your elbow on the inside of your leg. Curve your right arm over your head until it reaches your left foot, too (2). Carefully pull your left shoulder back to keep your body at right angles to the floor. Raise yourself gently then repeat on the other side.

1

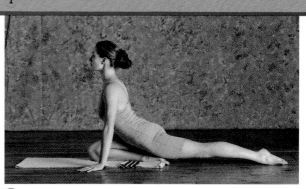

2

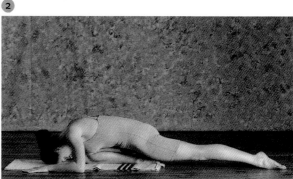

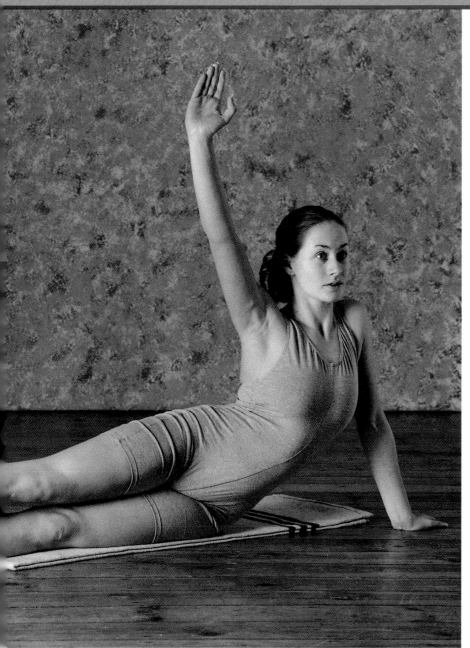

Dying swan
Resting on the floor on your hands and knees, extend your left leg straight behind you (1) and let your body follow naturally until your chest is resting on your right thigh. Keeping your head down and your arms relaxed, enjoy this position (2) for a few moments before beginning to use your arms to raise and lower your upper body, keeping your legs as they are. Repeat 10 times, then switch to the other side.

Sitting see-saw
Sit comfortably on the floor with your legs stretched out in front of you, ankles together and feet flexed. Place your left hand behind you on the floor for support, keeping the elbow straight, and rock gently onto your left hip, raising your right arm, elbow straight, above your head. Then rock over onto your right hip, raising your left arm in the air and lowering your right to the floor. Repeat 10 times on either side.

Legs and knees
targeted exercises

Day-to-day life is hard on our legs, because we deny them the chance for full and free movement. Instead, we spend too much time sedentary, sitting in unsuitable chairs, taking the elevator rather than the stairs or using the bus or train rather than the sidewalk.

Often when we sit, we do ourselves no favors. We cross our legs or we sit with them outstretched, both of which are bad for our circulation if nothing else. In the end, our legs lose their tone, and our knees become stiff and uncomfortable.

As with other parts of the body, freedom of movement and suppleness are what keep us young, slowing the ageing process. We need to maintain strong, toned legs and healthy knees simply to be able to walk, an obvious and everyday activity but one that is rarely practiced with the simplicity and grace it deserves.

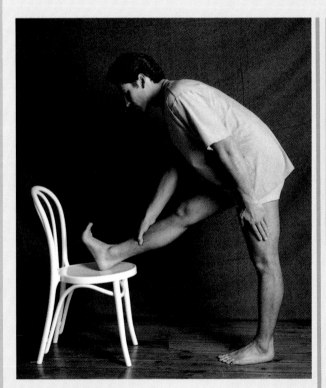

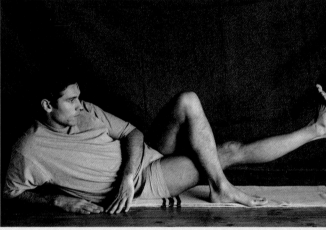

Knotted leg raising
Resting on the floor on your right side, use your elbow to support your upper body. Bend your left leg over your right, placing the left foot on the floor. Raise and lower your right leg, keeping it straight. Make sure you do not twist the right leg and that the rest of your body remains still. Repeat 15 times before switching to the other leg.

Standing hamstring stretch
Raise your right leg and rest your right heel on the seat of a chair, flexing your foot. Place your right hand on the top of your thigh and run your hand down toward your knee, keeping your back straight, your head up, and your foot flexed. When you feel a pull in the back of your thigh, hold for 10 seconds before repeating on the other side. Alternate legs until you have done four sets of 10.

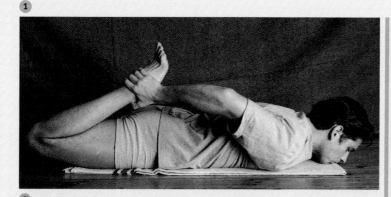

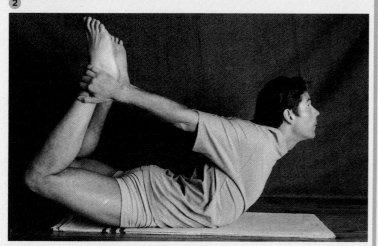

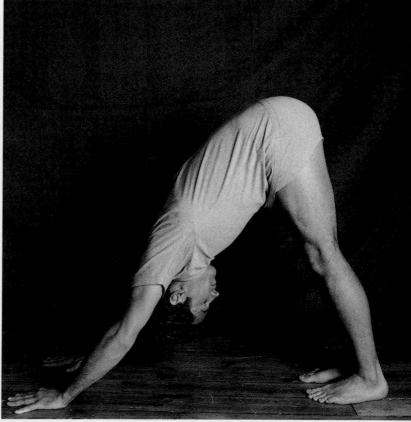

Bow pose and variations

Lie on your stomach on the floor, resting on your chin, with your hands by your sides. Bend your right leg at the knee and, reaching back with your right hand, grab your right ankle. Pull your heel gently as far as possible toward your buttocks, keeping your thigh flat on the floor (1). Hold this for 10 seconds, then relax and repeat on the left. Alternate left and right twice. If you find this very difficult, you can place a pillow or a folded towel under your thighs to raise them.

Once this is comfortable, you can achieve an even deeper stretch by lying on your side and working with your shoulders and back at the same time. Lying on your left side, bend both legs at the knee and reach down and behind to grab your right ankle with your right hand and your left ankle in your left hand. Pull your left foot up and away from your body. Hold for 10 seconds, then repeat on the other side.

When you feel strong and confident, you can move to the full position. Lying on your stomach, take hold of both ankles. Breathe in deeply, and as you breathe out raise your head and upper body at the same time as raising your thighs, so that your body curves (2). With each breath, try to rise a little higher, gently pulling against your feet to increase the stretch. Hold for as long as it is comfortable. Make sure you relax afterward – the full bow position is a formidable stretch for your entire body.

Mountain

This is a strong and difficult stretch, which will take some time to achieve fully. Standing with your feet parallel and separated at hips' width, bend over and put your hands flat on the floor about three feet in front of you. Push back with your arms, working to get your heels flat on the ground and your head toward the floor. Relax your head and neck letting them hang free. You will feel a deep stretch all along the back of your body.

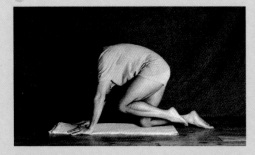

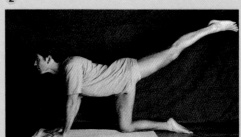

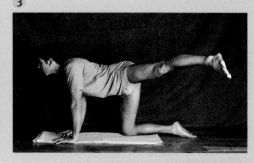

Rabbit kicks

Resting on the floor on your hands and knees, begin by arching your back upward. Looking down and lifting your left leg lightly off the floor, draw it under your body (1) to bring your left knee toward your forehead. Then, in a brisk movement, extend your left leg straight out behind you as high as it can go, at the same time as you raise your head (2). Repeat this 20 times, flowing the movements together, before switching to the right leg.

You can also kick out to the side. Again starting on your hands and knees, lift your left leg and extend it, knee straight, out to the side (3). Carefully kick up toward your shoulder, then back until it is straight behind you, trying to keep your body still by concentrating the movement in the leg. Repeat 20 times on the left, before switching to the other side.

Inclined plane

Sitting on the floor with your legs straight out in front of you, place your hands on the floor behind you, slightly wider than your shoulders, with your palms down and your fingers pointing toward your buttocks. Keeping your feet flat on the floor, raise your body from the ground until you create a flat plane from your shoulders through your feet to the ground. Hold for about 30 seconds, relax, and repeat. If you feel comfortable in this position, raise one leg and then the other to increase the stretch.

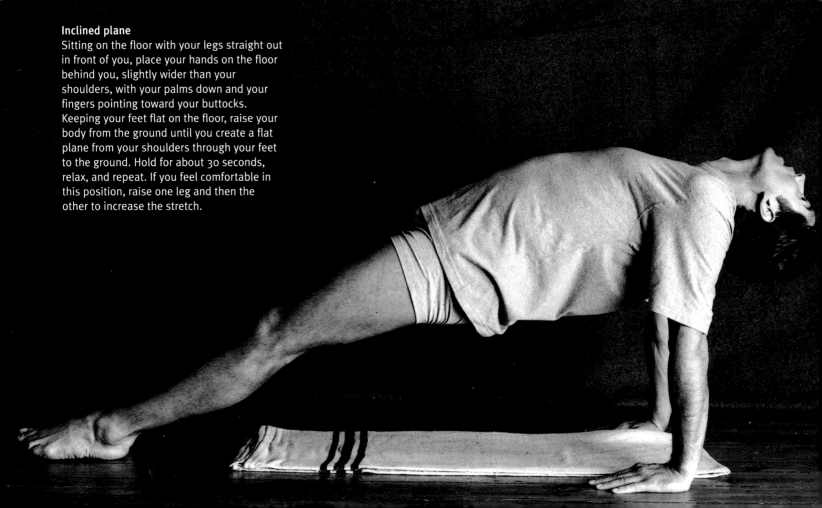

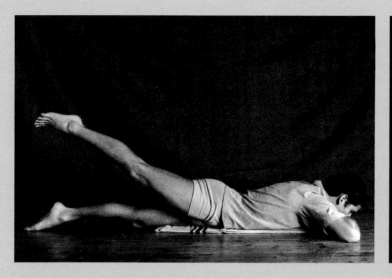

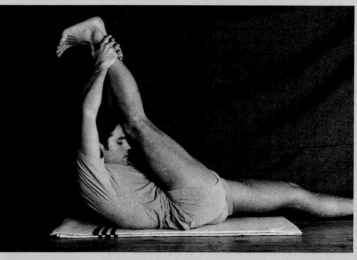

Leg raising

Lying on your stomach on the floor, bend your arms and place one palm on top of the other just in front of you, making a cushion for your chin. Keeping your right leg straight and your toes pointed, raise your right leg up into the air. If you think of lengthening the leg backward at the same time, it will help you to achieve a satisfying stretch. Slowly lower the leg to the floor and repeat 10 times before switching to the left leg.

Straight leg head to knee stretch

Lying on your back on the floor with your legs straight out in front of you, raise your right leg off the floor without bending your knee, and keep your left leg relaxed. Reach up and hold your right ankle with both hands, raising your upper body off the floor to do so. Bending your elbows, use the weight of your upper body to gently pull your right leg, working the hamstrings and the inner thigh muscles in particular. Hold this for about 30 seconds before releasing your leg and lowering it slowly to the ground. Rest and repeat on the other side.

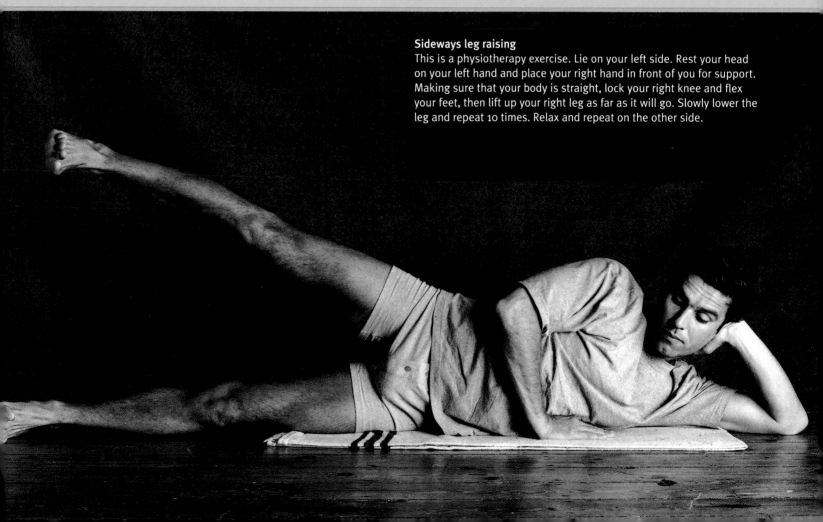

Sideways leg raising

This is a physiotherapy exercise. Lie on your left side. Rest your head on your left hand and place your right hand in front of you for support. Making sure that your body is straight, lock your right knee and flex your feet, then lift up your right leg as far as it will go. Slowly lower the leg and repeat 10 times. Relax and repeat on the other side.

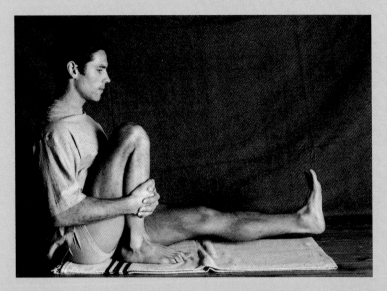

Sitting leg flex

Sitting on the floor with your legs straight out in front of you, bend your right knee and bring your right leg in close to your chest, holding it in your arms and keeping your foot on the floor. Then raise and lower your left leg five times with the foot flexed and five times with the foot pointed, before switching legs. Make sure you keep your back straight at all times, even if this means moving your upright leg away from your chest a little.

Half lotus forward bend

Sitting on the floor with both legs extended straight in front of you and your back straight, bend your right knee and place your right foot at the top of your left thigh. Gently push down at the right knee, trying to touch it to the floor. If this is too difficult, simply place your right foot on the floor as close to your groin as possible. When you are ready to take this a stage further, flex your left foot and, reaching down to take it in both hands, aim to touch your head to your left knee.

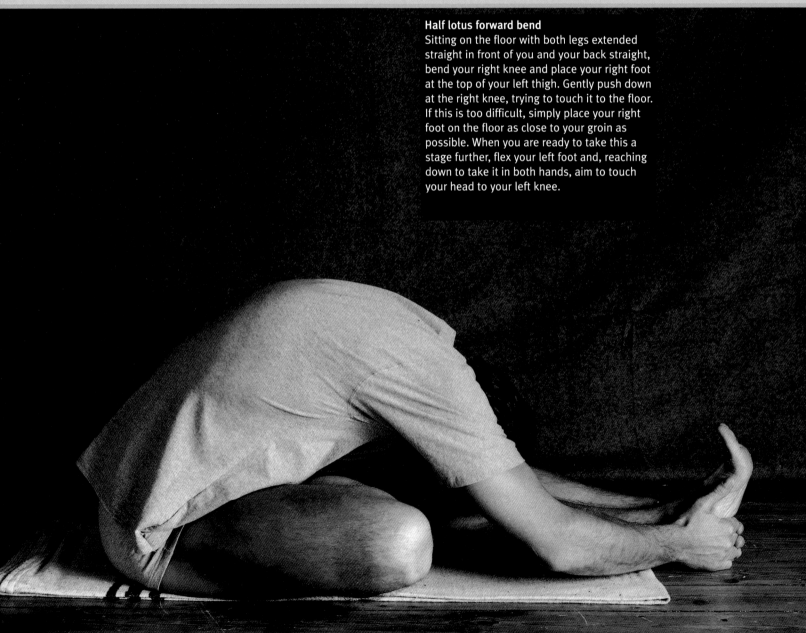

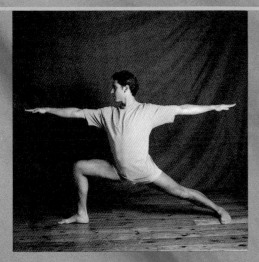

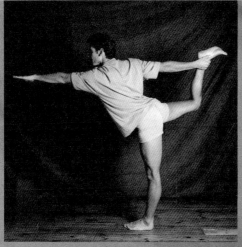

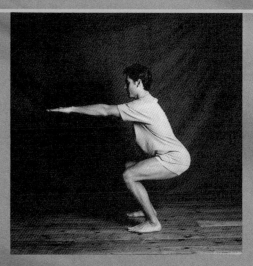

Warrior

This is a very powerful yoga position. Take your time and you will find it is a very deep stretch. Stand with your legs wide apart and your feet parallel. Turn your right foot 90 degrees to the right. Keeping your arms straight, stretch your hands out sideways, straight from your shoulders, as if you are being pulled in two directions. Turn your head to the right but keep your body facing forward.

Keeping your left leg straight and your left foot on the floor, bend your right knee until the right thigh is parallel to the floor. Make sure that your right knee remains in direct line with the heel of your foot.

Stare out over your right hand, making sure that your left leg is fully extended and in line with your hips. Hold this for 30 seconds before gently returning to your starting position and repeating on the other side.

Standing bow

Standing with your arms by your sides and your feet a few inches apart, raise your left arm straight up in the air. Bend your right leg at the knee and reach back to clasp your ankle with your right hand. Pull your right leg back, squeezing it against your hand. At the same time, stretch your left arm straight out in front of you. Hold your hips level and, keeping your head upright, fix your eyes on one point to help your balance. Hold this position for as long as you are able, then switch to the other side.

Chair squat

This is another example of how, sometimes, the simplest stretches can also be some of the most effective. Standing with your feet hips' width apart and your arms by your sides, bend your knees and lower yourself as if into an imaginary chair – but because there is no chair, your leg muscles must hold you in the sitting position. Raise your arms in front of you to balance. Remain like this for as long as possible. If this is very difficult, you can begin by propping your back against a wall, but if you do it this way, make sure your thighs are parallel to the floor and your shins are vertical.

Feet and ankles
targeted exercises

Think about the relief you feel at the end of a difficult day when you sit and take off your shoes, perhaps wiggling the toes to free them after their long confinement. This allows the feet and ankles the freedom of movement they were designed for. Your feet, small as they are relative to the rest of your body, manage to support your entire weight, distributed along the arches.

The toes grasp the ground, balancing and pushing off when we walk. By pivoting, the ankles provide balance and stability, and establish a hinge movement necessary for locomotion. But our shoes bind and constrict the feet and forbid the toes any range of motion; boots limit the movement of the ankles; and high heels force the front of the foot to bear more weight than it is designed for. So we develop flat, calloused feet and thick, stiff ankles – unattractive and uncomfortable.

The simplest way to do our feet a favor is to walk around without shoes for a while every day. The following stretches can also strengthen the feet and ankles, preventing injuries such as twisted ankles and fallen arches and making the feet more attractive.

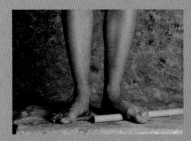 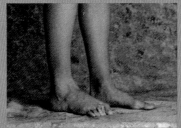 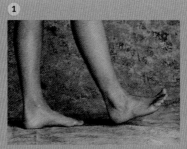 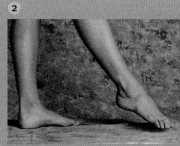

Stick massage
This will increase the circulation in your entire body and stimulate crucial nerve endings. It will also help you to improve your posture. Place a broomstick or a dowel on the floor. Starting with the left foot, rest your toes on the stick and press them down. Your feet will feel very sensitive, which is how it should be. Imagine you are breathing through your feet and the discomfort will ease. After a moment, roll your foot along slightly and press again. Continue in this way until you have worked your whole foot. If you can bear it, linger on the most sensitive areas, because they need the most massage. When you have finished the left foot, repeat with the right.

After rolling both feet, stand on the stick with your arches centered over it. Make sure you stand up straight throughout to gain the most benefit for your posture. Hold for as long as you can.

Foot massage and Foot wiggling
Often, from misuse, the toes have lost their strength and flexibility – think of the range of movement babies have in their toes. The first step to regaining this mobility is to stretch your toes with your hands.

Sitting comfortably, hold one foot in your hands. Take your big toe in one hand. Starting with the little toe, stretch it away from the big toe with the other hand. Pull each toe in turn. Then, one toe at a time, rotate each one gently.

One at a time, pull each toe backward, stretching the bottom of your foot; then do the opposite, bending your toes forward.

Then, sitting or standing with your feet parallel and about four inches apart, roll the feet outward, keeping your heels and the fronts of your feet firmly on the floor but lifting the arches (see picture above). Repeat this last exercise three times.

Foot rotation
You can do this in any position as long as you can raise one leg from the ground without tensing the rest of your body. Simply rotate one foot at a time from the ankle (1 and 2), five times clockwise and five times counterclockwise. Do not worry about a little quiet cracking sound, but make sure that you are turning your ankle gently enough so that you do not feel any discomfort.

Flexed foot kneeling
Kneeling on the floor, lean forward and support yourself with your hands as you turn your toes under so that the toepads are on the floor. When you are in this position, carefully shift back toward your heels, feeling a stretch in your toes as well as in your calves (see main picture on the opposite page).

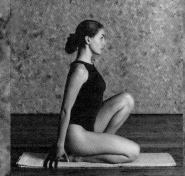

Heel press

Keeping your left leg bent for support, rest your right knee, shin, and upper side of the foot on a cushion or mat with the heel pointing straight up. Gently lower yourself so that your right buttock presses on your right heel, keeping your heel straight. Gently try to push down a little lower, and hold the stretch for at least 15 seconds. Relax, then repeat on the other leg. This will stretch the muscles on the upper side of the foot through the ankle to the front of the leg.

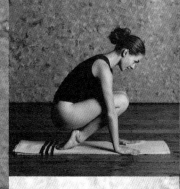

Toe squash

Kneeling on the floor with the tops of your feet flat against the ground, sit back on your feet. Put your hands on the floor beside you and push yourself, lifting your knees off the floor and rocking back onto your feet. You should feel a stretch along the outside of your ankles and along the top of your feet.

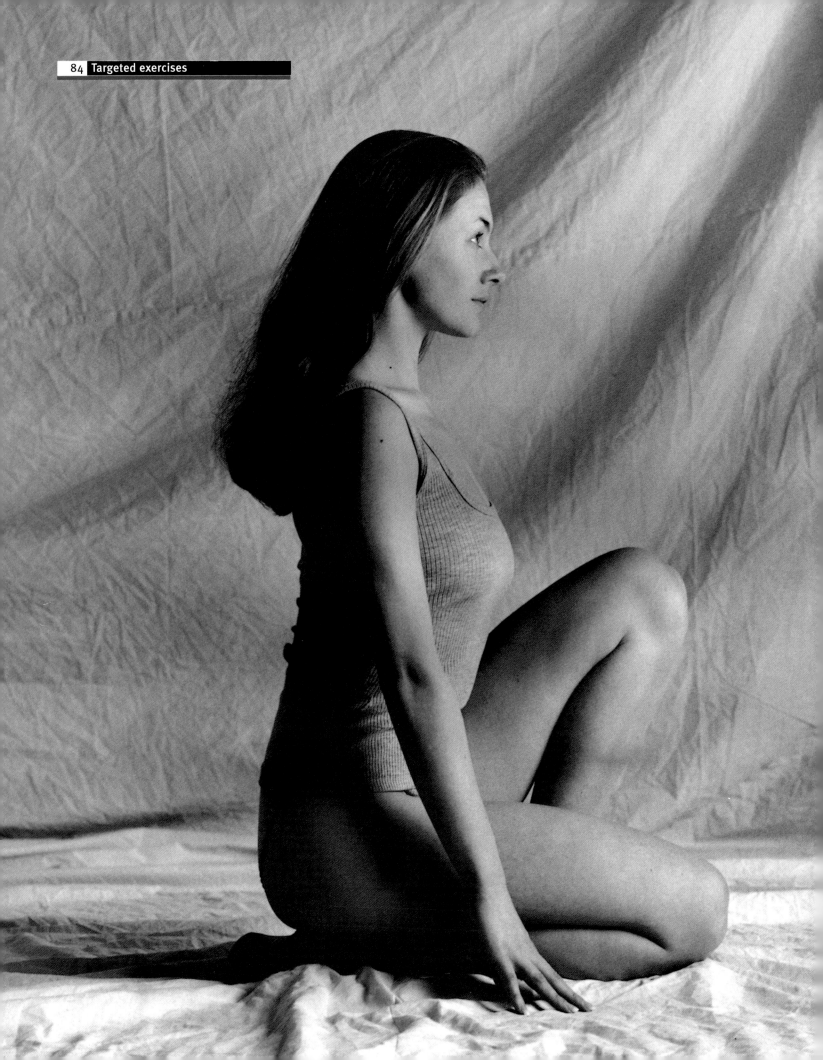

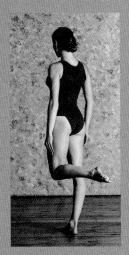

Flamingo
One of the most effective exercises for strengthening the ankles is also one of the simplest. Balance on one leg with your eyes fixed on one spot, or keep your eyes closed to make it more difficult. Aiming for stillness, try to hold your balance for at least one minute. It is harder than you may at first think.

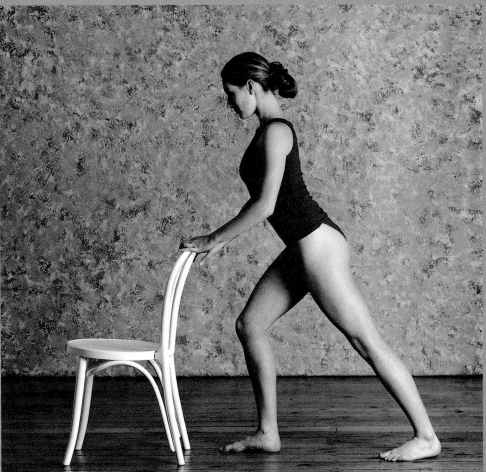

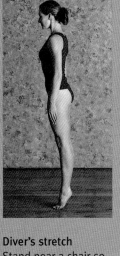

Diver's stretch
Stand near a chair so you can use the back of it to steady yourself if you need to. Keeping your feet close together and your ankles touching, raise yourself slowly up on your toes as high as you can. Hold this for as long as possible, then lower yourself slowly.

Tiptoes
Standing comfortably, with the back of a chair handy so you can use it for support if you want to, raise your right foot off the floor and hold it a little in front of you. Slowly raise yourself until you are balancing on your left toes, then lower yourself slowly. Make sure your ankles remain straight and that the sole of the foot doing the work does not turn in or out. Repeat twice, then switch feet.

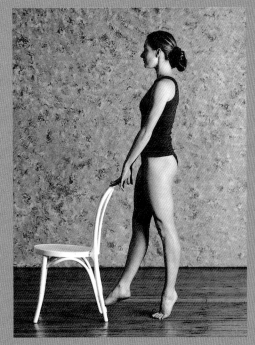

Achilles stretch
Leaning forward and supporting yourself against the back of a chair or the wall, place your left foot about 10 inches behind your right, keeping both feet parallel. Bend your right knee, keeping the right heel on the floor, and at the same time press your left heel down toward the floor, so you feel a gentle stretch along the back of your right calf.

Routines

Do not feel nervous about the idea of a regular routine – stretching for only 10 minutes a day will help you feel stronger and more supple. The key to a workout is to combine stretches that work different parts of the whole body from head to toe, incorporating a warm-up and cool-down. Eventually, your body will grow so used to daily stretching that you will wonder how you ever lived without it.

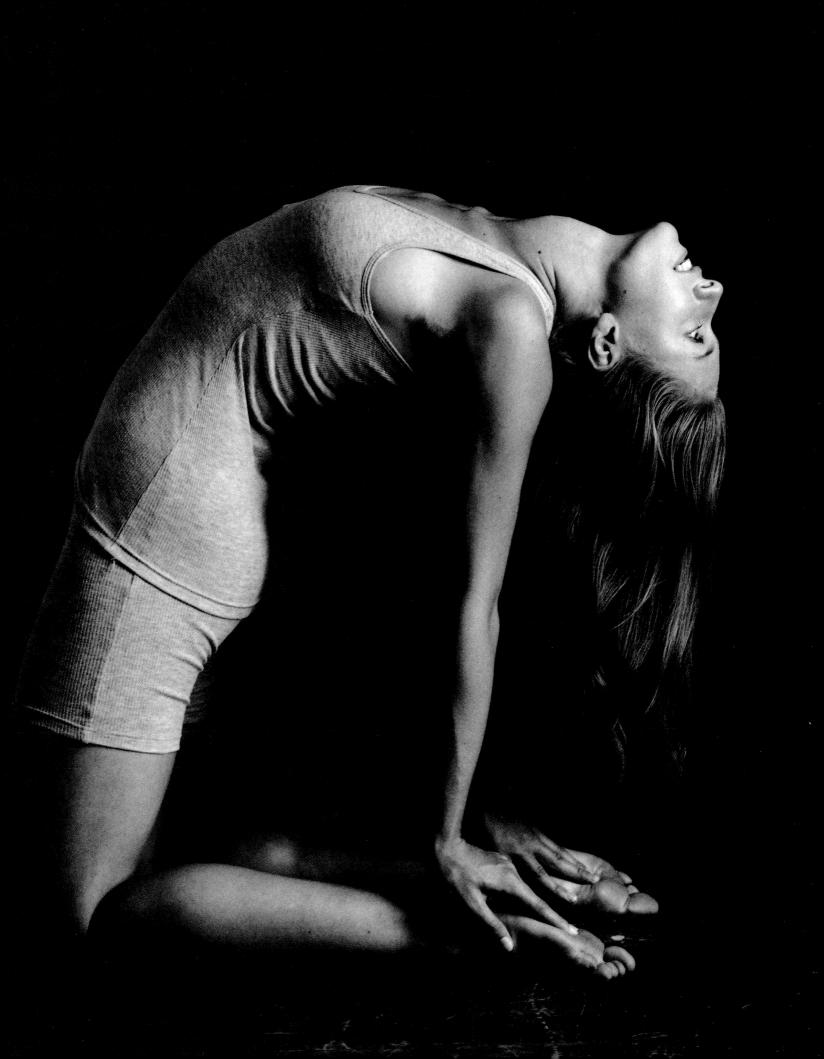

Routines general advice

Ultimately, the only way to become fitter is with practice. By now, you should be developing a clearer picture of the state of your health, fitness, and flexibility, but the only way to achieve lasting improvement is to take what you have learned and use it in a regular routine. A daily workout does not need to be as daunting as it may sound. In fact, you will find that it can be both a soothing and an enjoyable part of your day-to-day life.

For the best results, you should think of doing at least a short routine every day. The exercises in this book are not the type that require you to wait a day or two before repeating them. In fact, the more you do them, the better you will feel and the more comfortable you will become with the idea of doing a routine. Once your body has become accustomed to daily stretching, you will wonder how it was that you ever managed without it.

The big question always is: where do you find the time? This is why you will see three different routines, starting with one that lasts only 10 minutes (no excuses possible with this one) through to one that lasts half an hour. As the routines get longer, the level of difficulty also increases. The timings, however, are just guidelines: the 20-minute routine may take you a little less or a little more time than that.

As you become more experienced, you may want to create your own routines, either concentrating on areas of your body that you particularly want to work on, or catering to a certain mood or circumstance in your life. It may be easiest to begin by customizing the routines in this book, substituting some of your favorite exercises for others. But eventually you can create your own routine from scratch. On the opposite page are a few guidelines that will help you to design routines that work well.

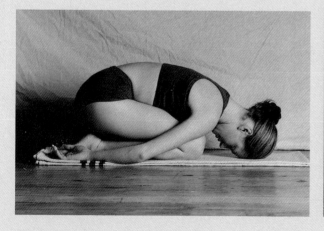

Child pose, page 92

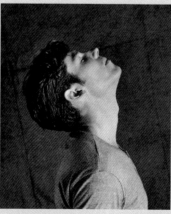

Head cross, page 94

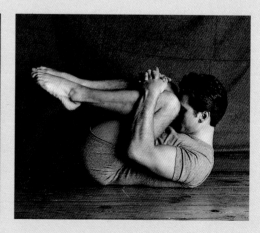

Head to knee roll, page 97

Once you have devised your routine, don't change it too often. Ultimately, you want it to become so familiar that you can relax and listen to your body without the distraction of worrying about either the sequence of exercises or how to do them correctly. This way, by the end of the routine, you will not only be physically healthier but also mentally refreshed.

1 Each routine must incorporate a warm-up. For example, the head cross or gentle stretches at the beginning of the following routines are perfect warm-up exercises.

2 The routines that you decide on should be structured so that they follow a logical pattern, with one stretch flowing smoothly into another.

3 It is sensible to group exercises so that, say, all the standing stretches are done together, followed by all the sitting ones.

4 Choose for yourself just what you want to achieve with the routine. You can emphasize fitness or suppleness or combine the two. Basically the sky is the limit.

5 Finally, it is essential to remember not to force things – always work at your own pace and comfort level.

10 minute routine

Ideal for the beginner, but equally useful for those more experienced, this is something that you can do as you tumble out of bed in the morning, as you prepare for the day ahead – or last thing in the evening, maybe after a hot bath. In fact some of the exercises can even be done while you are still in bed.

A simple 10-minute routine is not designed to build up strength or stamina, but rather to encourage you to unlock your body, either after the stresses of a long day or after the inactivity of a night's sleep. This is why it is important to remain relaxed and to remember that it is quality, not quantity, that counts.

Bear in mind, especially if you are doing this first thing in the morning, to keep it gentle. Listen to the signals that your body is giving out, and don't push too hard. Breathe deeply and relax. You will find that one stretch flows into another.

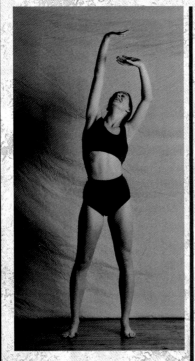

Gentle stretching
This is something that is easily done while you are still in bed in the morning. Raise both arms above your head and stretch, first with your right arm and then with your left (1). You should feel your body lengthening, especially your back. As you breathe out, reach a little higher. Do this five times on each side. If you want to get out of bed, this exercise can also be done standing up.

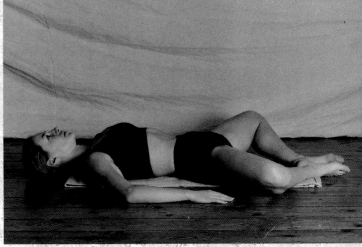

Lying butterfly
This is as it sounds. Lie on your back on the floor with your knees bent and your heels touching. Drop your knees as far apart as possible (2). To keep your lower back straight, you may want to tilt your pelvis upward slightly, which will push your back into the floor. Relax and hold for around 45 seconds, breathing deeply.

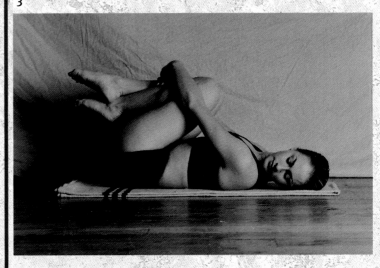

Cradle
Lie on your back on the floor, lift both your knees and, clasping them with your hands, pull them toward your chest. Relax and gently rock, turning your head to the left as your legs move right and vice versa (3). Continue to rock gently for about one minute.

4

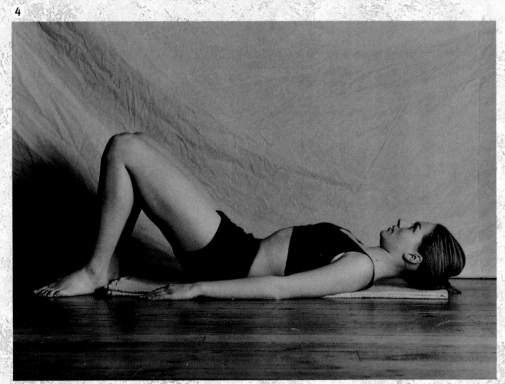

Abdominal tilt
Lie on your back on the floor with your knees bent and your arms resting at your sides (4). Without raising the lower back, gently lift the pelvis by working the stomach muscles. Relax and lower the pelvis back down to the floor. Repeat 10–20 times.

5

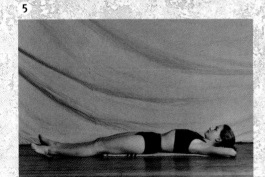
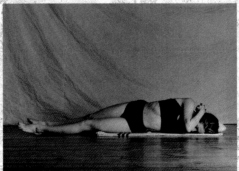

6

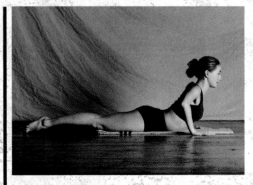

Lying twist
For the upper spine. Clasping your hands behind your head, let your elbows flop flat on the floor. Keeping your heels on the ground, turn your upper body to the left, trying to touch your right elbow to the floor next to your left elbow (5). Hold this position for around 15 seconds before relaxing and turning the other way. Repeat.

Simple push-ups
Lie on the floor on your stomach with your legs straight behind you and your palms on the floor by your shoulders. Raise your upper body, letting your arms do most of the work, keeping your pelvis on the floor (6). To complete this exercise, lower yourself again, supported by your arms. Repeat 10 times.

7

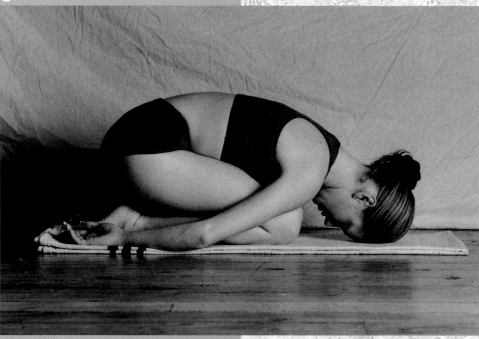

9

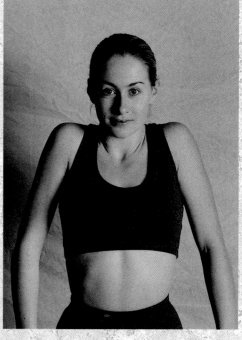

Child pose

This is a traditional yoga position, which is both calming and comfortable. Kneeling, with your buttocks resting gently on your feet, bend over until your head rests lightly on the floor, and place your arms by your sides with your hands resting, palms up, by your feet (7). Hold this position for around 45 seconds – a break after the exertion of the last few exercises.

8

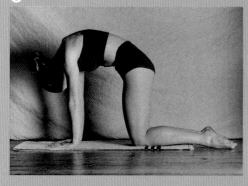

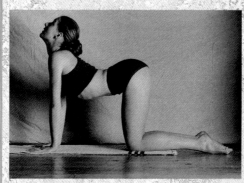

Cat arching

Kneeling, with your hands on the floor directly under your shoulders, arch your back upward to hunch it and drop your head. Then curve your back in the opposite direction to hollow it, at the same time raising your head up (8). Do this about 10 times each way.

Shrug

As you breathe in, raise your shoulders up toward your ears (9) as high as you can. Hold them there for five seconds, then, as you breathe out, let them drop freely. Relax and breathe out again and, as you do so, think of relaxing your shoulders a little more. Don't try to force them, because the simple power of suggestion will be enough to let your shoulders release that little bit more. Repeat five times.

10

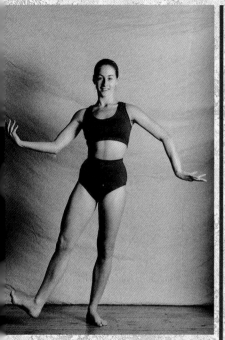

11

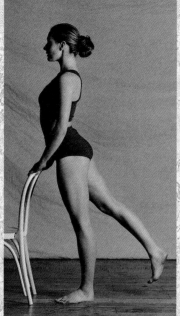

12

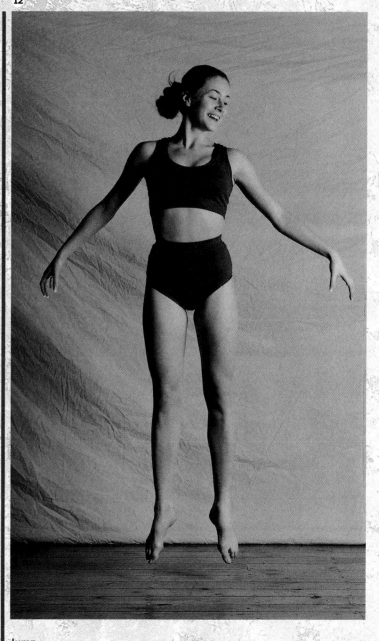

Foot and hand rotations
Rotate your ankles and your wrists, five times in a clockwise direction and five times counter-clockwise.

Chair aerobics
Stand behind the chair with your feet hips' width apart, holding lightly onto the back for balance. Keeping your right leg straight, lift it to the right, with your foot facing forward. Repeat five times before raising it behind you, again keeping it straight (11). Repeat in this direction five times before switching to the left leg.

Jump
This is a nice way to round off. Jump freely and lightly up in the air a few times to release any final tension and to feel fresh and rejuvenated.

20
minute routine

It doesn't take a major time commitment to work toward greater fitness and flexibility. If you consider that an average television sitcom is longer than 20 minutes or that it takes about that time to skim through your morning paper, you will realize that a regular, thorough work-out won't eat into a busy lifestyle.

This is a little more vigorous than a simple warm-up, but it shouldn't leave you too tired to take on the other challenges in your day. Remember to start slowly and work into the routine gently, and you should find that one exercise leads naturally into the other. A few minutes concentration on these exercises should clear your mind of life's worries and leave you feeling positive and alert.

①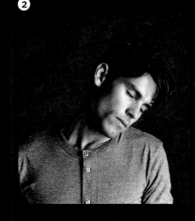

②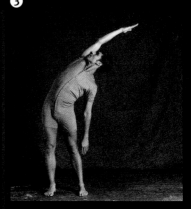

③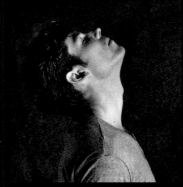

Gentle stretching
Stand with your feet hips' width apart. In turn raise each arm above your head and stretch toward the ceiling, first with your left (1) and then with your right. You should feel your body lengthening, especially your back. As you breathe out, reach a little higher. Do this five times on each side.

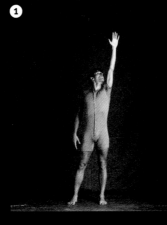

Head cross
Drop your head forward until your chin is resting on your chest. Slowly raise it then lower it to the left, aiming to touch the ear to the shoulder (2). Then lower to the right, again aiming to touch the ear to the shoulder. Finally, look up toward the ceiling. Keep your shoulders still and level and let your jaw hang loose. Do this three times.

Crescent stretch
Keeping your feet flat and hips' width apart, raise your right arm and bend slowly over to your left, without bending forward or backward at the waist. You should feel a strong stretch all along your right side. When you are comfortable, turn your head up slightly (3). Hold for 20 seconds then switch sides. Repeat twice on each side.

④

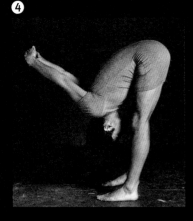

⑤

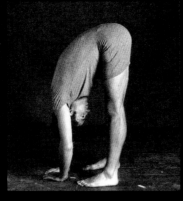

⑥

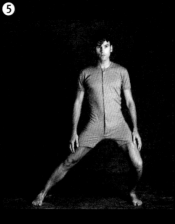

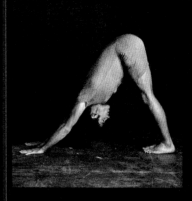

Clasped hand forward bend
Standing with your legs hips' width apart, clasp your hands behind your back, interlacing your fingers with your palms facing up. Bend forward from the waist, letting your arms follow naturally. You should feel a stretch not only along the back of your body, especially your legs, but also in your shoulders. Then release your hands, letting your arms dangle in front of you (4). Nod your head gently in little yes's and no's, feeling a release in your neck. Hang there for at least 30 seconds, then slowly curl up to the original standing position.

Sideways groin stretch
Standing with your feet two or three feet apart, bend your left knee, feeling the stretch in your right inner thigh (5). Make sure you keep your body upright. Hold for around 15 seconds, then reverse the stretch.

Mountain stretch.
Standing, feet hips' width apart, bend over and put your hands flat on the floor about three feet in front of you. Push back with your arms, working to get your heels flat on the ground and your head toward the floor. Release your head and neck and let them hang free (6), feeling a deep stretch along the back of your body. Hold for 30 seconds.

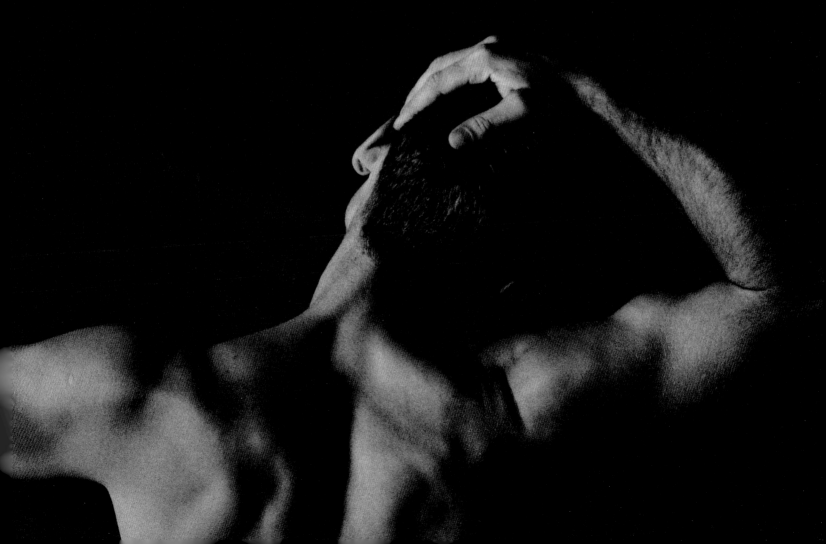

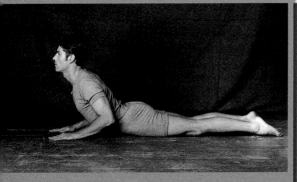

Cobra stretch

Lying on the floor on your stomach, place your hands flat on the floor with your thumbs level with your armpits. Raise your head up slowly, arching your back (7). Do not use your arms to push – rather let your back and your abdomen do the work. Hold this for 10 seconds then try to rise a bit higher for 10 seconds more. Relax and return your body to the floor.

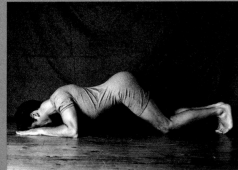

Caterpillar

Lie on your front on the floor with your chin resting on the floor and your hands, palms down, by your armpits. Drop your forehead until it touches the floor, relax your upper body, and, lifting your pelvis and lower back (8), slowly drag yourself back until your head approaches your knees and your buttocks rest on your heels. Try to keep your forehead on the floor and your hands where they started. Rest for a moment in this position, known as the child pose (see page 92), before releasing your hands and curling up into a kneeling position.

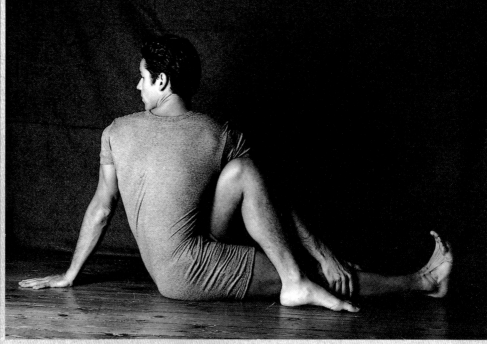

Sitting spinal twist

Sit on the floor with both legs straight in front of you and your spine upright. Pick up your left leg and, bending the knee, put your foot down on the right side (outside) of your right knee. Put your left hand on the floor behind your left buttock, without bending your elbow. Lift your right arm and, keeping the elbow straight, bring it over your upright left knee and place your right hand lightly on your right leg. Turn and look as far as you can over your left shoulder, thinking of raising your lower back (9). Hold for 30 seconds, release and switch sides.

10

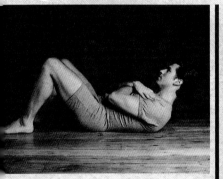

11

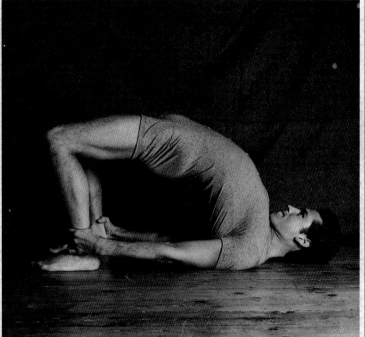

12

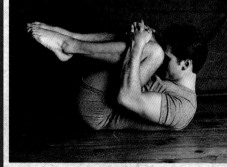

Curl ups

Lie on your back on the floor with your knees bent and your hands lightly crossed on your chest. Keeping your lower back on the floor and your neck aligned with your spine, use your abdominal muscles to raise your upper body off the floor, starting with your head then your upper trunk, but take care not to lift your lower back (10). Slowly lower yourself to the starting position. Repeat 15 times. Be careful not to rush.

Bridge pose

Lie on your back on the floor with your knees bent and your feet hips' width apart. Reach down and hold your ankles – if you can't reach, place your palms flat on the floor with your arms extended. Lift your pelvis, trying to raise it as high in the air as possible (11). Hold for 30 seconds, return slowly to the floor and repeat.

Head to knee rolls

Lying on the floor, bring your knees in to your chest and raise your forehead to touch your knees (12). Rock gently from side to side for 30 seconds.

13

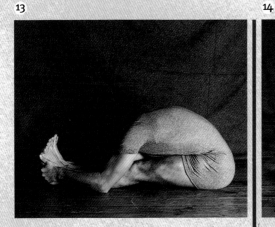

14

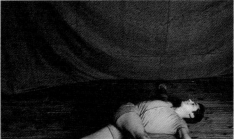

15

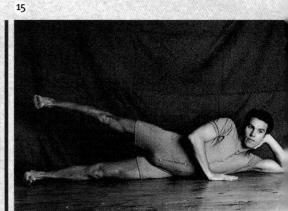

Forward bend

Sit upright on the floor with your legs stretched straight out in front of you and your feet flexed. Waddle your buttocks back a little to make sure you are sitting on your hip bones. Reach straight up, stretching your arms high above your head, and bend over from your waist, aiming to take hold of your toes (13). Relax and stay in this position for about a minute before releasing. Curl back slowly, one vertebra at a time, until you are lying on your back.

Lying spinal twist

Lying on your back on the floor, raise your right leg up and over your body, lowering it to the ground on your left side, keeping your shoulders flat on the floor (14). Hold for 30 seconds before switching to the other side.

Sideways leg raising

Lie on your left side on the floor. Rest your head on your left hand and place your right hand in front of you for support. Making sure that your body is straight, lock your right knee and flex your feet, then lift your right leg up as far as it will go (15). Slowly lower the leg and repeat 10 times. Relax before doing the exercise on the other side.

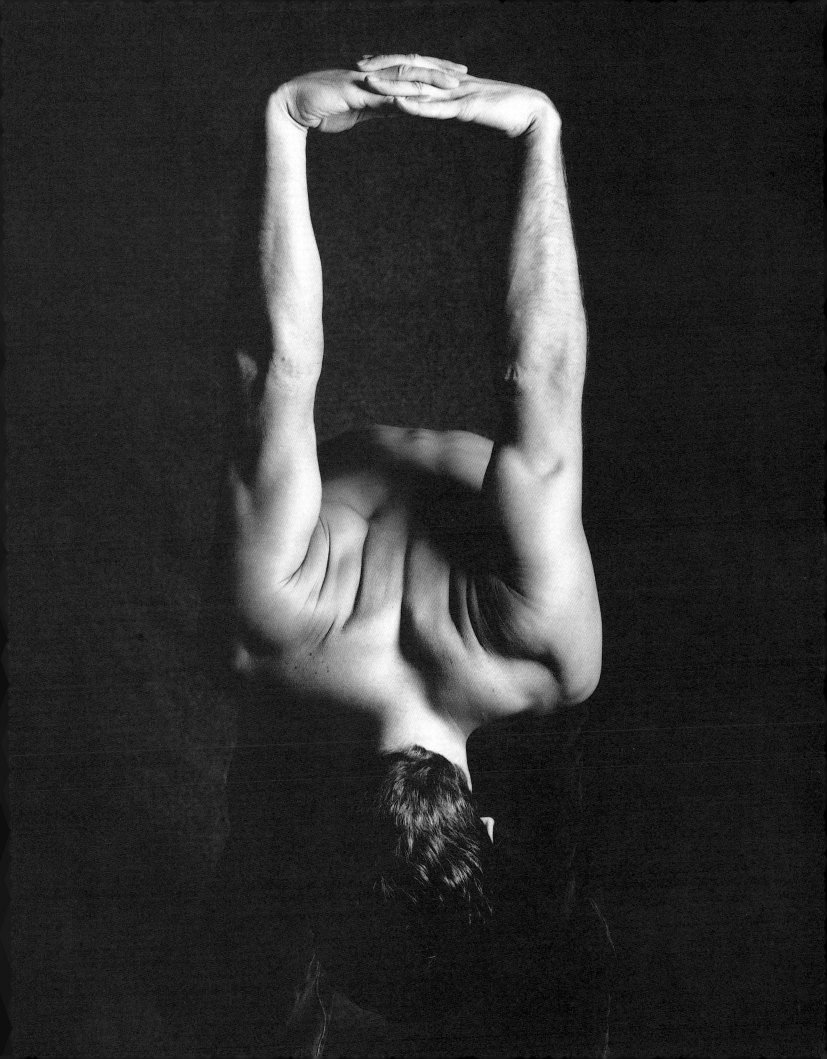

30

minute routine

While the briefer routines are designed to squeeze a regular workout into a busy schedule, spending a little more time is ultimately more rewarding. Not only can you increase the number of exercises you do, but the extra time lets you concentrate completely on what you are doing and gives you the opportunity to include more advanced and intricate stretches.

As always, begin slowly and work your way gently into the routine. Like the others, this routine is designed so that one exercise flows into another, but you will find that it is more strenuous and advanced than the early routines. For this reason it is advisable not to eat a heavy meal before doing it. Also you will want to leave yourself a little time at the end to relax and cool down.

Take your time and relax into the routine. It won't be long before it becomes so satisfying that half an hour will seem like a very short time indeed.

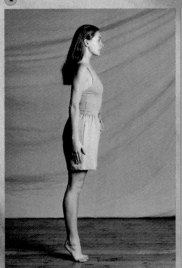

①

Diver's stretch, shoulder roll, and head cross
These are three good warm-up stretches. For the diver's stretch, keep your feet together and ankles touching, and raise yourself slowly up on your toes as high as you can (1). Use a chair to steady yourself if you need to. Hold for as long as you can and lower yourself slowly.

Next, stand with your arms relaxed by your sides. Raise one shoulder toward your ear. Rotate it slowly forward then down, then back and up again toward your ear, keeping the movement as full and circular as you can. Do this three times in each direction, then change sides, keeping the rest of your body as still as you can.

For the head cross, keep your jaw loose and shoulders level. Drop your chin onto your chest. Slowly raise your head and lower it to the right, aiming to touch the ear to the shoulder, then lower it to the left in the same way. Now look at the ceiling. Repeat twice.

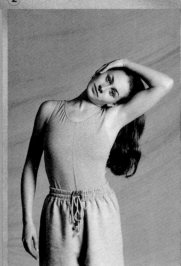

②

Sideways head clasp
Standing or sitting, tilt your head to the left, so your ear approaches your shoulder. Reach up with your left arm and hold your head, with your palm cupped over your right ear (2). Relax your left arm so its weight exerts a gentle pull. To enhance this stretch, keep your right arm horizontal, flexing your hand at the wrist. Hold for 20 seconds, release and switch sides.

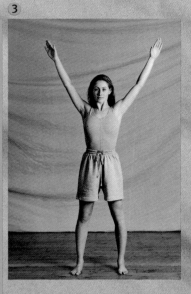

③

Stick 'em up
A position you will have seen in countless westerns, this is a marvelous exercise for your shoulders and pectoral muscles.

Stand with your feet hips' width apart and your arms raised above your head as if you were a surrendering soldier (3). Keeping your arms straight and your palms facing forward, push your arms back behind you as far as they will go, before returning to the starting position. Do not be surprised if this movement is not very big, but you should feel a pull across the top of your chest. Flap back and forth in this manner 20 times before resting, and then repeat the whole sequence twice more. Remember to keep your shoulders down and your neck long.

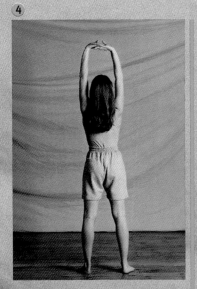

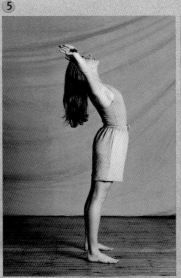

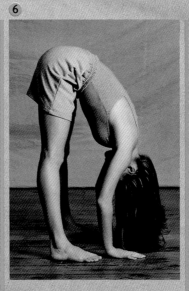

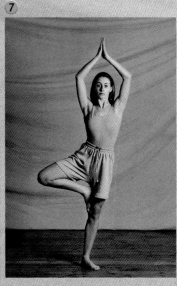

Tower

Standing comfortably, interlock your fingers and, with your palms facing up, stretch your arms above your head (4). Make sure your elbows are straight and your upper arms are pulled behind your ears. Relax and breathe, thinking about stretching up through your back. Hold for about 30 seconds before resting and repeating twice more. Reclasp your fingers each time with a different thumb on top.

Backward bend

Separate your feet a little wider than your hips for better balance, and place your palms on the backs of your thighs. Tightening your buttocks and pushing your pelvis out in front or you, stretch backward as far as you can, letting your hands slide down your thighs. Let your jaw open. You should feel the stretch both in your upper back and in your abdominal muscles. Hold for 20 seconds and straighten up.

When you feel confident with your balance and your back is more supple, you can do this bend with your hands raised over your head (5).

Forward bend and hang

Standing with your feet hips' width apart, tip over from the waist and, without locking your knees, reach down to your feet (6). It should feel like your upper body is hanging down from your hips. Keep your weight evenly spread across your feet and, with each breath, relax your stomach muscles and let your back get looser. Relax in this position for around 30 seconds, then return to the backward bend. Alternate these two exercises twice more.

Tree

Begin standing with your feet together. Lift up your right foot and place the sole of that foot on the inside of your left thigh. Reach down and, using your hands to help you, bring your foot as high up your thigh as possible. Place your palms together in front of your chest and, keeping them pressed together, slowly raise your hands above you so that your palms are above the crown of your head. Keep your neck long and your shoulders down (7).

Now, fixing your gaze staight in front of you to help your balance, straighten your arms so that your upper arms touch the sides of your head, keeping your palms together. Relax and aim to hold this position for a minute before slowly returning your hands to chest level and placing your right foot back on the floor. Repeat on the other side.

8

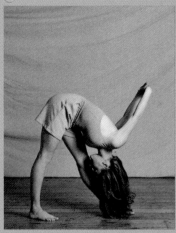

9

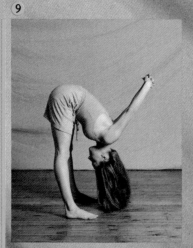

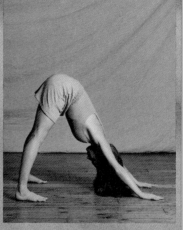

10

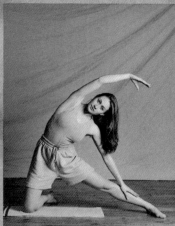

Clasped hand head to knee bend
Place your left foot about two feet in front of you. Clasp your hands behind your back, interlacing your fingers with your palms upward. Bend forward from the waist, letting your arms follow naturally until your forehead touches your left knee or is as close to it as you can get (8). Keep this position for 30 seconds, relaxing your shoulders, thinking of touching the floor in front of you with your hands. Return to the starting position, relax for a moment, switch legs, and repeat.

Clasped hand forward bend in triangle (9)
Standing with your legs as wide apart as they can comfortably go and your feet facing forward, clasp your hands behind your back, interlacing your fingers with your palms facing up. Bend forward from the waist, allowing your arms to follow naturally so that they swing forward as far as they can go without straining. You should be able to feel a stretch not only running along the back of your body, but especially in your shoulders. Then release your hands and place them on the floor in front of you, pressing back in order to increase the stretch.

Finally, place your hands on the backs of your calves and try to pull your body closer to your legs. Keep your balance in this position as you relax for a moment before uncurling slowly.

Kneeling crescent moon
Kneeling upright on the floor, extend your left leg out at a right angle to your body. Without twisting your upper body, raise your right arm and stretch it up and over your head toward your left foot. Meanwhile, slide your left arm down your thigh toward your foot (10). Hold for 30 seconds then repeat on the other side.

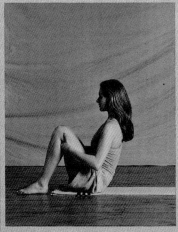

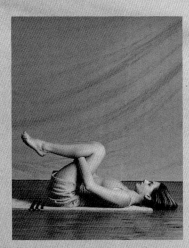

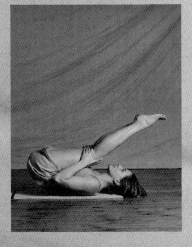

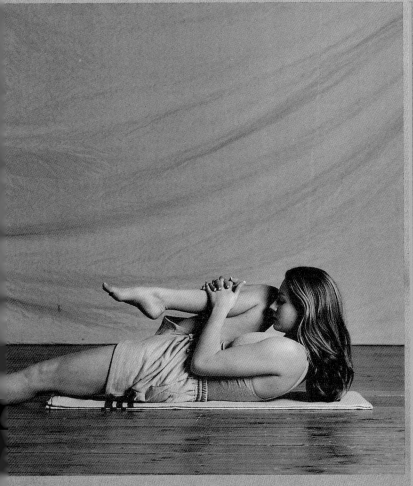

Head to knee stretch

Begin by lying on the floor. Clasping your right knee with your hands, pull the knee toward your chest. Lift your head and try and touch your knee with your forehead. To enhance the stretch you might like to try and touch your knee with your nose or ear (11). After about 30 seconds, relax and repeat on the other side.

Spine rolling (12)

This is an excellent way to release the whole of your spine. Lie on the floor with your legs in the air and your knees bent. Gently hold the backs of your thighs just beneath your knees. Now relax and pull your knees toward you so that you roll backward, aiming to touch your knees to your forehead. You may find it more comfortable if you straighten your legs as you roll backward. When you have rolled back as far as you can go without straining, breathe out and then roll forward as far as you can, allowing your knees to flop open into a butterfly (see page 104) and your head to approach the floor.

Roll backward and forward in this way for about a minute, breathing in as you roll backward and out as you roll forward. Be gentle and you will find this very relaxing. As a variation, you can cross your ankles and clasp your big toes as you roll. This will give a deeper stretch and particularly help you to release your neck.

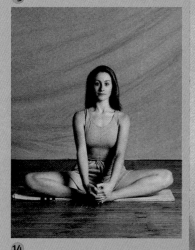

Butterfly

Sit on the floor with your knees bent and the soles of your feet touching. Hold your feet with your hands and pull them as close to your groin as you can without slouching in the lower back (13). The aim is to get your knees to touch the floor, so gently push down on your thighs with your elbows or lightly bounce your knees up and down. Hold for between one and three minutes and relax. If you have enough time and you feel like it, you can add some variations (see page 70).

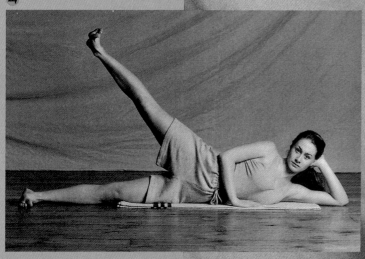

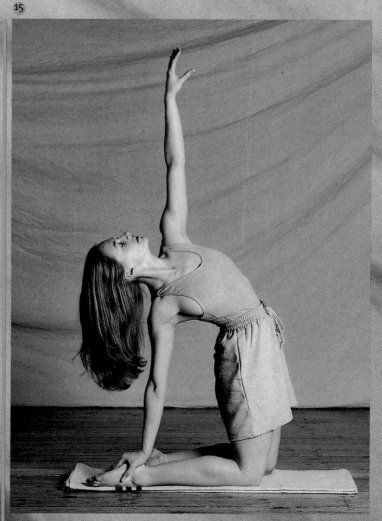

Sideways leg raising

Lie on your left side on the floor. Rest your head on your left hand and place your right hand in front of you for support. Making sure that your body is straight, lock your right knee and flex your feet, then lift your right leg up as far as it will go (14). Slowly lower the leg and repeat 10 times. Relax and repeat on the other side.

Camel with twist

This is an advanced backward bending stretch. Kneeling up on the floor with your legs a little wider than hips' width apart, gently reach back and place your left hand on top of your left foot, keeping your pelvis up and facing forward. When you are comfortable and balanced, carefully lower your right hand so it is on top of your right foot and drop your head back. Keep your buttocks squeezed together so your lower back is not strained.

For a stronger stretch, push forward with your hips. When you are comfortable, raise your left arm and hand straight up in the air and turn to look up at your hand (15). Breathe deeply and hold for 30 seconds before switching arms.

If you have time for a variation, try this: place your right hand on top of your left foot, dropping your head back. When you are comfortable, raise your left hand. Look down at your foot, hold, relax and breathe deeply.

16
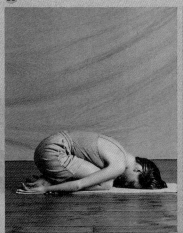

17
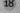
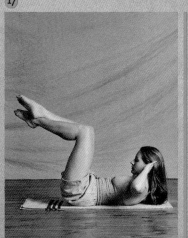

18
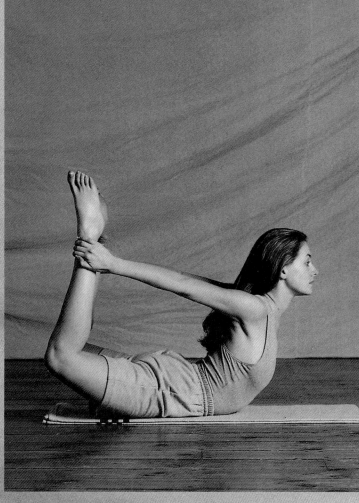

Child pose

This is a traditional yoga position, which is calming and comfortable. Kneeling, with your buttocks resting gently on your feet, bend over until your head rests lightly on the floor. Place your arms by your sides with your hands resting, palm up, by your feet (16). Hold this position for around one minute – a period of rest after the exertion of the last few exercises.

Crunchies

Remember with these to keep your lower back on the floor and keep your neck in line with the spine.

Lie on the floor with your fingers gently touching behind your ears. Lift your legs and, bending your knees at 90 degrees, cross your ankles. Then, without jerking, lift your head toward your knees until you feel a pull in your stomach (17). Relax back down and repeat 10–20 times, recrossing your ankles in the other direction halfway through. Remember how many you have done and do three more sets of that number.

Bow pose

Lying on your stomach, reach back and hold both ankles on the outsides. Breathe in deeply and, as you exhale, raise your head and upper body at the same time as your thighs, so that your body curves (18). With every breath, try to rise a little higher, gently pulling your feet to increase the stretch. Hold the position for 20 seconds without straining too much. Relax and repeat twice more.

The following relaxation will let your breathing settle and your mind clear before you get on with your day. Lie on your back on the floor with your legs straight and hands resting, palms up, by your sides. Close your eyes and remain in this position for three minutes.

In the office
routines

Anybody who works regularly in an office can testify to the aches and pains that come from spending a lot of time sitting at a desk, not to mention the mental and emotional stresses of competitive office environments. But there are, thankfully, a number of ways to counteract the physical discomforts of working in an office, where normally the only exercise you take is a walk to the filing cabinet and back again.

There are some inconspicuous but highly effective stretches you can do anywhere and any time, without your colleagues thinking you have gone crazy. Some stretches are done when you are sitting in your chair, while others, like the Office Squat or the Toe Stand on page 108, can be done while you are looking for papers in a filing cabinet or books on a shelf. If you type a lot, you can also find some relief for your hands in the hand massages suggested on page 48.

Even if you cannot do some of these exercises every day, remembering to sit up straight in your chair and to get up and walk around a little bit every half hour or so will help prevent so many of the all too familiar discomforts of office life. The key is to keep in mind that exercise is as much a part of your day-to-day life as your work is, and if you are feeling fit and relaxed, your work will only improve.

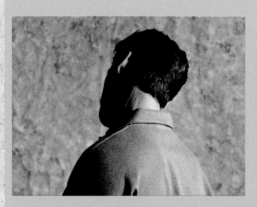

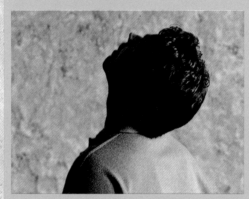

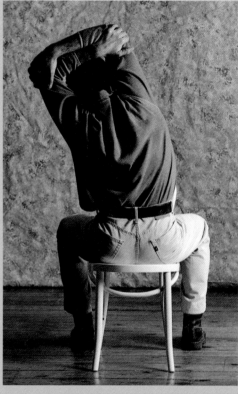

Head cross
Your neck suffers greatly from the stresses of the day and it is important to take time to relax it. As is often the case, one of the most effective ways is also the simplest. Sitting comfortably, let your head drop forward, bringing your chin toward your chest. Breathe deeply, feeling a release in your neck and down your back. Slowly raise your head, then drop it sideways so that your right ear approaches your right shoulder, but be careful not to raise your shoulder (1). Again breathe deeply, before raising your head to center again (2) and allowing it to drop toward your left shoulder.

Elbow clasp side bend
Sitting upright and relaxed on a chair with both feet flat on the floor, raise both arms above your head and clasp each elbow in the opposite hand. Pull your upper arms as far behind your ears as possible. Keeping your elbows high and back, bend your upper body slowly to the left. Relax and breathe. Hold for about 10 seconds and then repeat on the other side. Aim to stretch at least three times on each side.

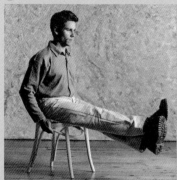

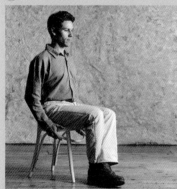

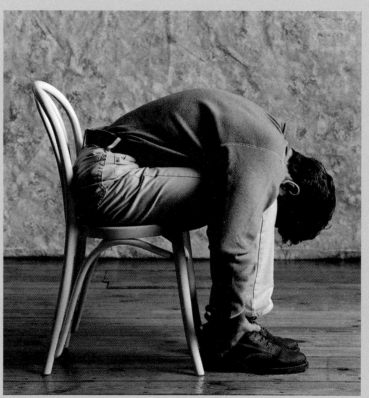

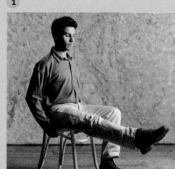

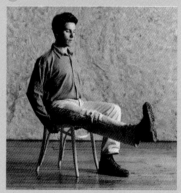

Ankle twist

Sitting comfortably in a chair, put your legs straight out in front of you. Cross your legs at your ankles, right over left (1), and squeeze one ankle against the other, holding for five seconds then releasing for five seconds. Repeat 10 times, then switch so that the left ankle is over the right. You can also do this exercise with your feet on the floor (2). Aim to increase the amount of time you spend squeezing, building up to as much as 30 seconds.

Chair forward bend

Sitting comfortably in a chair with your feet flat on the floor, bend forward and hold on to your ankles, consciously relaxing your neck and shoulders.

Foot flex

Sitting comfortably in a chair with your feet flat on the floor, raise your right leg, extending it straight out in front of you (1) and flex and point your right foot 10 times (2), before lowering it gently and switching to the left.

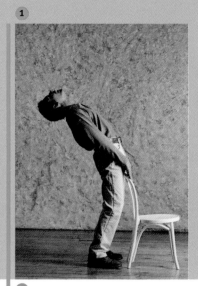

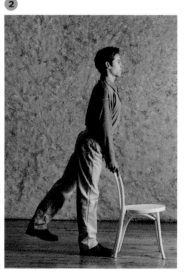

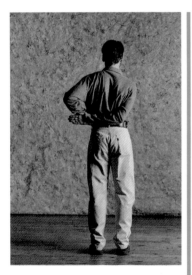

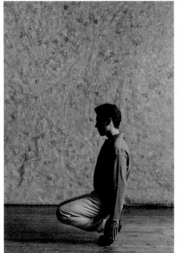

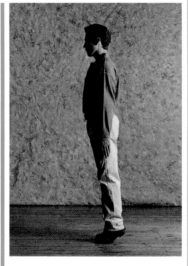

Hand cuff stretch

Reaching behind you, take your right wrist in your left hand and pull it across to the left, keeping your body still and upright. Hold for 15 seconds and then repeat on the other side.

Office squat

This is a balance as well as a stretch, which works your whole leg from ankle to thigh. Bend down from your knees, balancing on your toes and keeping your knees together. Aim to hold your thighs parallel to the floor. Balance for 30 seconds, then stand up slowly. If you need to, support yourself against a wall or a piece of furniture.

Toe stand

From a squatting position balancing on your toes, stand up straight, remaining on your toes the entire time. It sounds simple, but it actually demands a surprising combination of strength and balance.

Chair aerobics

Stand behind a chair with your feet hips' width apart. Holding lightly onto the back of the chair for balance, bend your knees slightly and allow your pelvis to tilt forward, gently curving your lower back (1). Straighten up and then repeat five times.

Keeping your left leg straight, lift it to the left, with your foot facing forward. Repeat five times before raising it behind you, again keeping it straight (2). Repeat in this direction five times, before switching to the right leg.

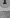

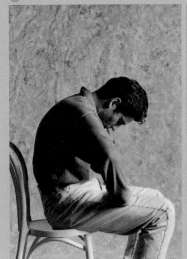

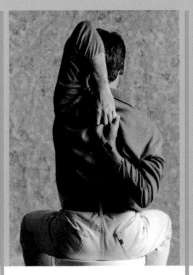

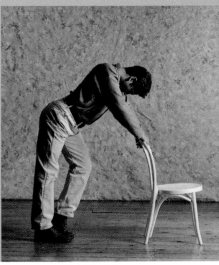

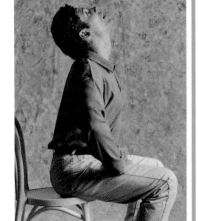

Sitting back roll

Sitting comfortably in a chair with your feet flat on the ground and your arms by your side, allow your head to drop and slump down as far as you can (1), breathing out and releasing tension throughout the length of your back. Then, breathing in, straighten up as much as you can (2). Repeat 10 times.

Chair twist

Sitting in a chair with your feet flat on the floor, twist to the right to face behind you. You can brace yourself by nestling the left side of the seat in the crook of your right elbow if possible, but if you cannot reach, just hold the seat back any way possible and use it to pull yourself gently into a deeper twist. Hold, breathing deeply for as long as you are comfortable, then release and relax before twisting in the other direction.

Cowface

Sitting comfortably on the chair with your feet flat on the floor, raise your left arm above your head, perhaps using your right arm to tug it gently up a little higher, so that the left side of your body is stretched. Bend your left elbow, so your forearm is lowered behind your head. Holding your left elbow with your right hand, gently nudge your left arm a little lower, increasing the stretch in your shoulder, but making sure the right elbow points up. Bring your right arm around and clasp hands, or, if you cannot quite reach, hold onto your shirt. Hold this position for around 30 seconds, or as long as it is comfortable. If this is very difficult, just repeat the first stage. Switch arms and repeat.

Mime strut

Standing in front of your chair, about a foot away, and bend over to place your hands firmly on the seat of the chair. Alternatively, stand behind your chair and place your hands on its back if this is more comfortable for your height. Bend your left knee and your left toe, extending your right hip slightly out to the side, then slowly shift your weight and position, until your left toes and your right knee are bent and your left leg is straight. It will look a bit like the way a mime artist pretends to walk. Repeat this 15 times. You should feel action in your legs and hips and a relaxation of your lower back.

Duos

Working with someone else, such as your partner or your child, adds a new dimension to gentle stretching. It encourages trust and inspires new confidence in yourself and in your partner. You learn to cooperate, sharing the feelings of well-being. Most importantly, working together, with its companionship and contact, is highly enjoyable.

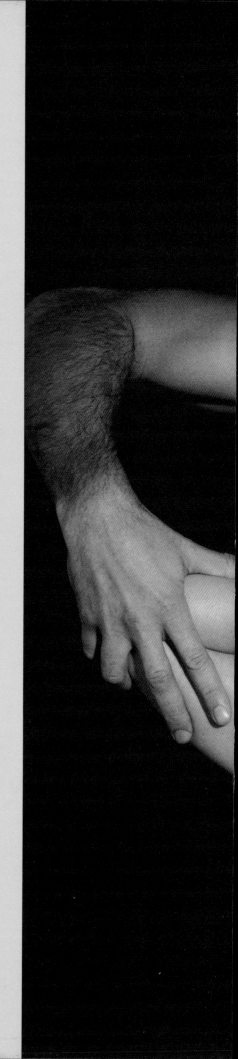

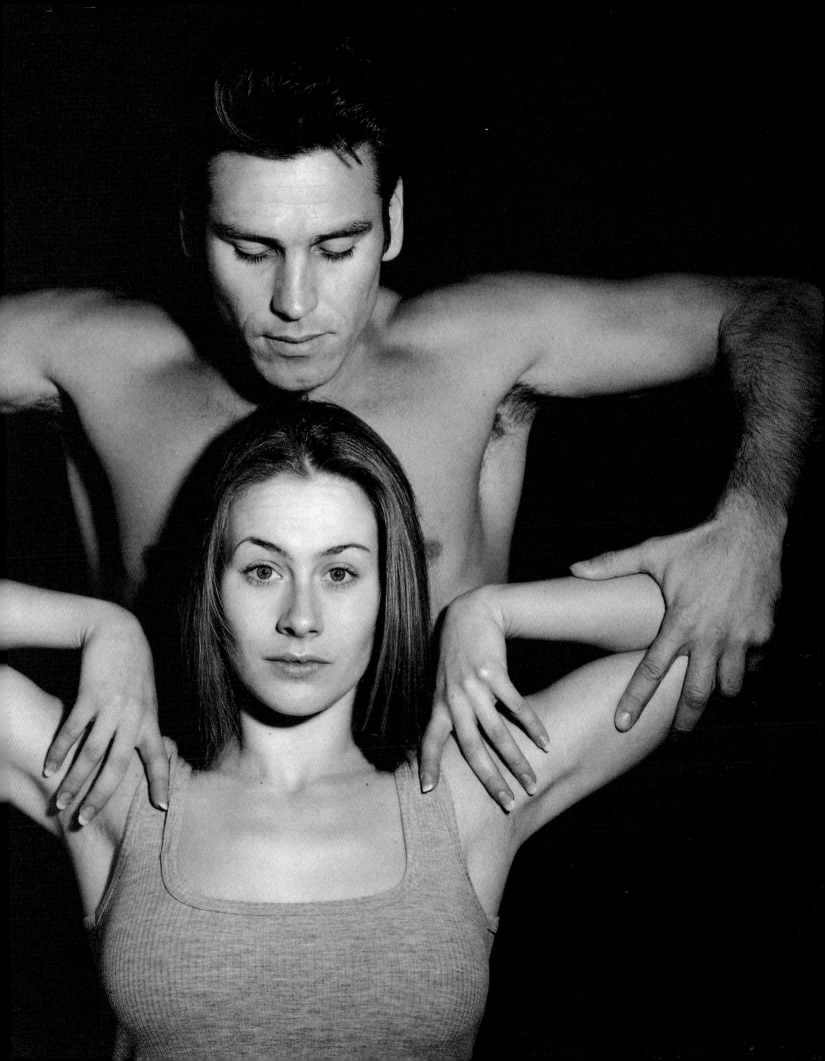

Duos general advice

Working with someone else – your child or your partner – adds a new dimension to exercise. It may feel a little uncomfortable at first, because working together requires trust on many different levels.

First we have to come to terms with how we see ourselves. Because we are led to believe that there is a perfect body that only the lucky few can achieve and maintain, we can easily develop a negative self-image. When you are exercising, your attention – and your partner's – is focused on your body, and you may feel exposed and vulnerable. This is part of the reason many people find it difficult to exercise in front of others.

Another reason is that, despite our best intentions, an element of competition can come into play. It is easy to make comparisons – "the other person can reach higher, they can hold the pose longer." This also can make us feel less secure.

Finally, in working together, there is a dependency involved. You have to be confident that your partner will not hurt you, and your partner has to have that same confidence in you.

The solution to all these anxieties is trust. You must trust that your partner is not judging you, and trust that you can put the other's best interests first. And you must communicate, responding to each other's bodies and moods.

The benefits of working together are infinitely rewarding. Because the physical body is so closely connected to the mental state, the trust that you must have with a partner to work together will also strengthen your emotional relationship with that person.

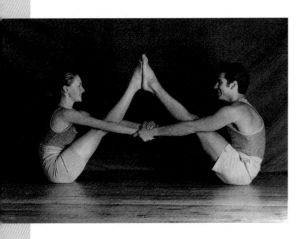

Drawbridge stretch, page 115

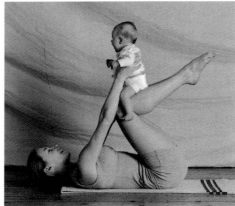

Shin rock, page 122

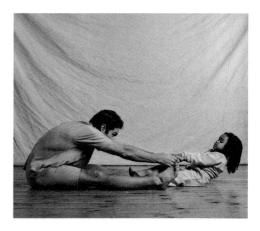

See-saw, page 125

The exercises that follow generally require physical contact, but this is not the only way to work together. Try going through a routine together without physical contact, just keeping each other company. You may choose to do the stretches one at a time, with your partner encouraging you and checking that you are doing the exercise correctly, and then switching roles. It is helpful to have someone point out things that you could never spot on your own, even if you are working with a mirror.

1 As always, take time to warm up. Each of you should devise your own warm-up – although if you are working with your child, it may be best to make suggestions.

2 Begin gently. Start with simple stretches first, and do not push your partner too far – or let yourself be pushed beyond what you feel is comfortable.

3 Make sure that you are both familiar with the exercises, understanding what you are going to do before you begin.

4 Always remember that you are not in competition. Ultimately, only you can decide how far each stretch should go.

5 Listen to your body – and your partner's. Pay as close attention to your partner's moods and body as you do to your own.

With your partner
duos

As your knowledge and flexibility develop, it is very satisfying to participate in exercises with a partner. Many Eastern relaxation techniques, such as t'ai chi, require a partner not only because working with another person is one of the best ways to test our strength and suppleness, but also because the gentle maneuverings and physical adjustments necessary to reach a shared goal mirror the ebb and flow of personal relationships.

In doing these exercises, it is very important to relax and enjoy yourself. Most of the stretches require no more than the gentle shifting of the body's weight, and the movement is often very subtle. By breathing deeply, trusting your partner, and relaxing completely, you will be able to tune into each other's bodies, and it will become easier to gauge each other's needs. Sometimes, the expression on your partner's face will tell you everything you need to know. And if you feel like laughing, go ahead – it will help to release unwanted tension.

Above all else, bear in mind that each body is unique, and only you know what feels right and what hurts. By remembering at all times to communicate with your partner, you will find that you can achieve deeper stretches, more advanced exercises, and have fun at the same time.

Shoulder drop
This is almost more of a massage technique than a stretch, and it is very effective in releasing a lot of the hidden tension that we keep trapped in the area of the neck and shoulders.

Stand behind your partner, who must relax completely, like a rag doll (1), and agree to let you do all the work. Gently take hold of your partner's upper arms and lift them so that the shoulders rise up toward the ears (2). When they can go no higher, release and drop them. It is very important that you are the only one doing the lifting – you will be able to feel whether or not your partner is totally relaxed. Repeat this five times before changing roles.

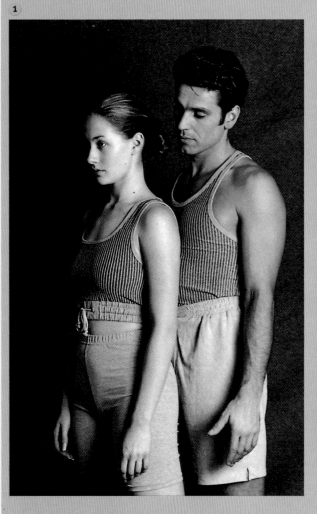

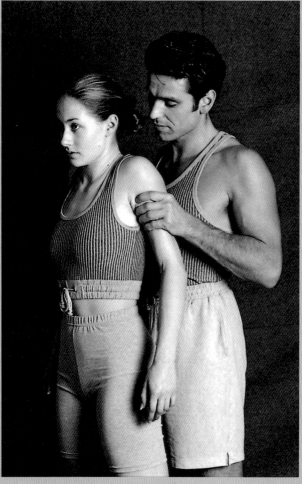

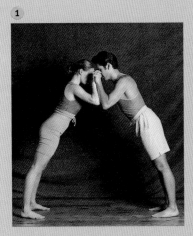

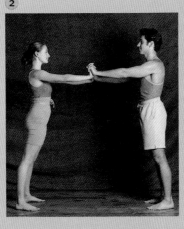

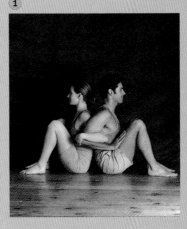

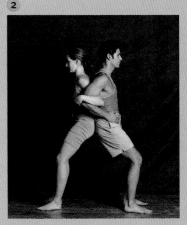

Standing push-ups

This is just as it sounds. Stand facing each other with your palms together and fingers clasped at shoulder height, with your elbows bent (1). Push back against each other as you straighten your arms (2), then return to the center. Repeat 20 times.

Suspension bridge

This exercise is a lot of fun – don't be surprised if at first you dissolve into laughter. Sitting on the floor with your backs together and your knees bent in front of you, interlock your arms at the elbows (1). Take a breath and as you breathe out, push against the floor and each other to raise yourselves up into a standing position (2). Rest at the top before reapplying the pressure and gently returning together to a sitting position. Repeat five times.

Drawbridge stretch

Begin by sitting on the floor facing your partner with your legs straight out in front of you, your knees slightly bent and the soles of your feet touching. Reach forward and take hold of your partner's wrists. With your head up and back straight, press against one of your partner's feet. Working together, lift that foot up into the air, each of you straightening your leg and keeping the soles together. Do not let go of your partner's wrists or you will both tumble backward. Hold for 10 seconds then return the foot to the floor and repeat on the other side.

Finally, press against both feet and lift both legs into the air at once. You will make a shape reminiscent of raised drawbridge. Remember to keep lifting in your lower back, and don't let go until you have returned your feet to the floor. Hold for one minute if possible.

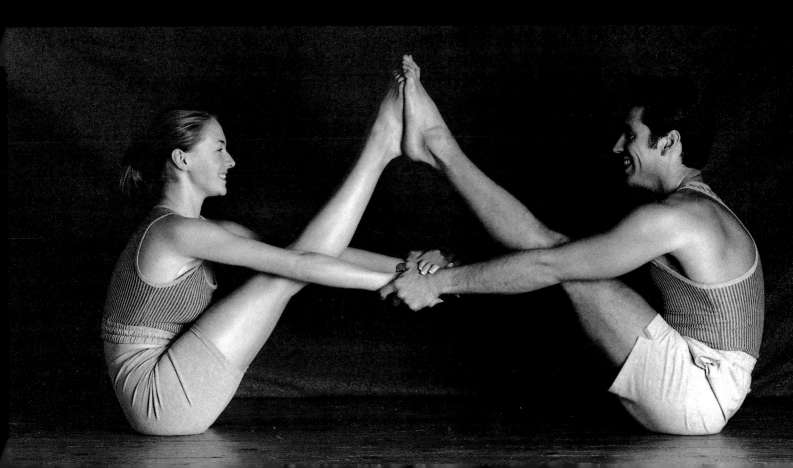

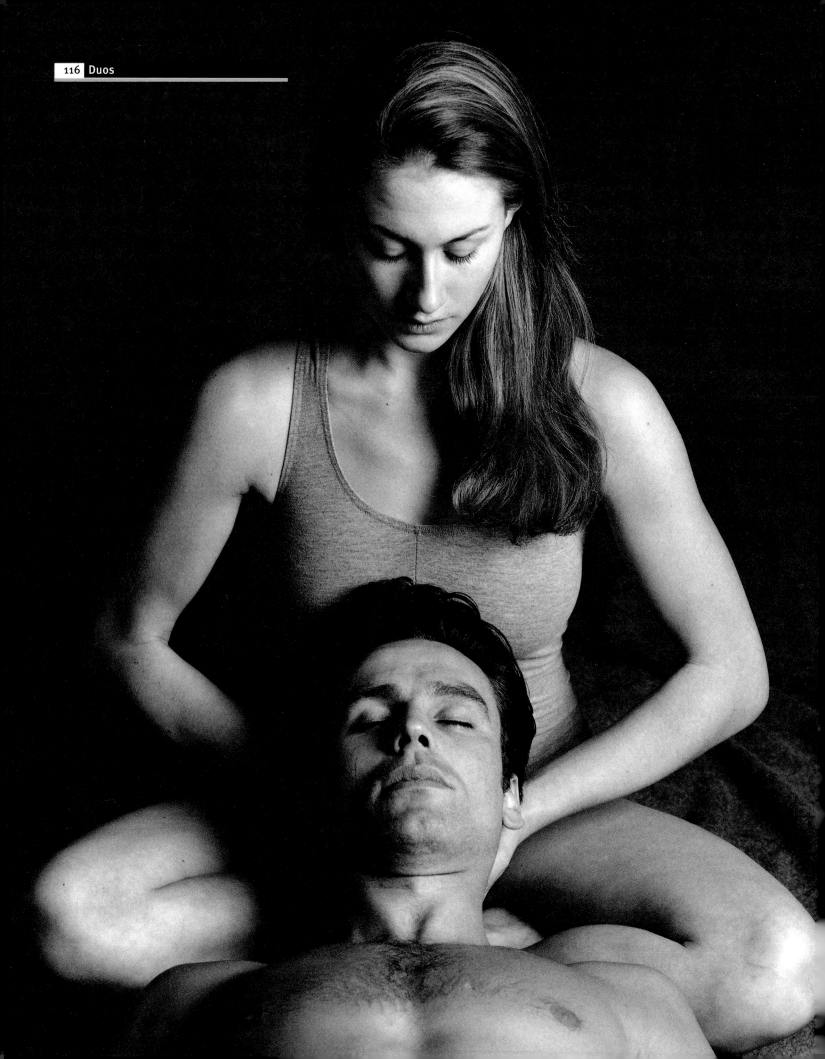

Head holding for two

To begin with, decide with your partner who is going to be the pulled and who the puller.

The pulled: Lie on the floor on your back with your knees bent and pointing to the ceiling and your hands resting lightly on your hip bones. Close your eyes and relax completely, trusting your partner and breathing deeply.

The puller: Sit or kneel on the floor just behind your partner's head. Rest your hands under the head and slowly take its weight in your hands, lifting it about an inch off the floor (see picture on opposite page). The head should feel very heavy – if it does not, encourage your partner to trust you and let you take the whole weight of the head.

From this point there are a number of things you can do. You can start by gently pulling the head away from the shoulders: holding the head firmly in your right hand, stroke your partner's neck with your left and as you do so pull gently, feeling the neck lengthening. When your left hand meets your right hand, carefully switch the weight of the head to the left and repeat. Then, holding the head in both hands, lift it up until the chin rests on your partner's chest. Hold for a few seconds, then return the head to the start position an inch off the floor. Finally, gently turn the head slightly from left to right a few times before slowly returning it gently to the floor. Relax and switch roles.

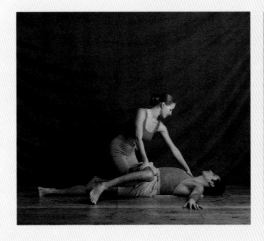

Partnered lying twist

Lying on the floor on your back, raise your right leg up and over your body. Bending your knee, lower it to the ground on your left side, paying attention to keeping your shoulders flat on the floor. Relax completely and now let your partner do the work.

The partner: Kneel on the right side of your partner, at hip level. Place your left hand on your partner's right shoulder and your right hand on the right knee. Push the knee and shoulder down to the floor, listening carefully to your partner's body and not pushing too hard. When your partner has had enough, relax and do the other side before switching roles.

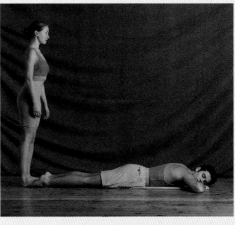

Foot-to-foot massage

Lie on the floor on your stomach with your arms by your sides. Relax and breathe deeply.

Partner: Stand directly behind your partner's feet. Now gently rest the ball of your right foot on your partner's right instep, then rest the ball of your left foot in your partner's left instep. Your heels should remain firmly on the floor so that your partner's feet do not bear all your weight. Shift your weight slightly, swaying from side-to-side and back-and-forth, massaging your partner's feet with the balls of your own. Continue for as long as is comfortable for both of you, then switch roles. It is normal to feel a tingling in your feet for a while afterward.

Feet press

Sit on the floor facing each other with your legs apart and extended in front of you. Place your feet inside your partner's and try to push your partner's legs apart as they offer resistance. Keep this up for about 30 seconds, then your partner can try to push your legs in as you offer resistance. Again, keep this up for around 30 seconds before switching roles.

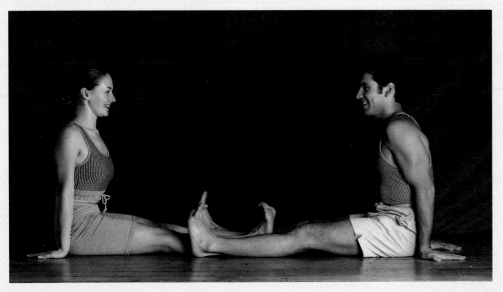

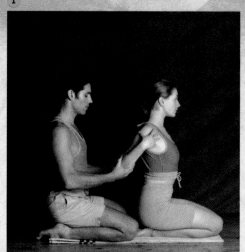

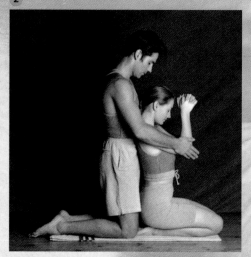

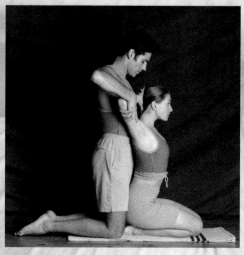

Backward shoulder pull

Kneel upright behind your sitting partner, who places their hands on their shoulders. Your partner must relax completely and agree to let you do all the work.

Reach forward and gently take hold of your partner's elbows. Pull them back, squeezing them together gently until they are touching (1). Encourage your partner to relax and enjoy the stretch, varying the intensity of the pull. To relax those muscles once the stretch is finished, gently push your partner's elbows in front (2). Rest and switch roles.

Partnered elbow pull

This is a strong stretch for your shoulders and upper back. Again, decide which of you will be pulled and puller.

The pulled: Sit cross-legged on the floor, placing your hands lightly on top of your head.

The puller: Kneel upright behind your partner. Take the partner's elbows firmly in your hands, pulling them gently back and wrapping them around your torso. Hold for as long as is comfortable. Relax and switch roles.

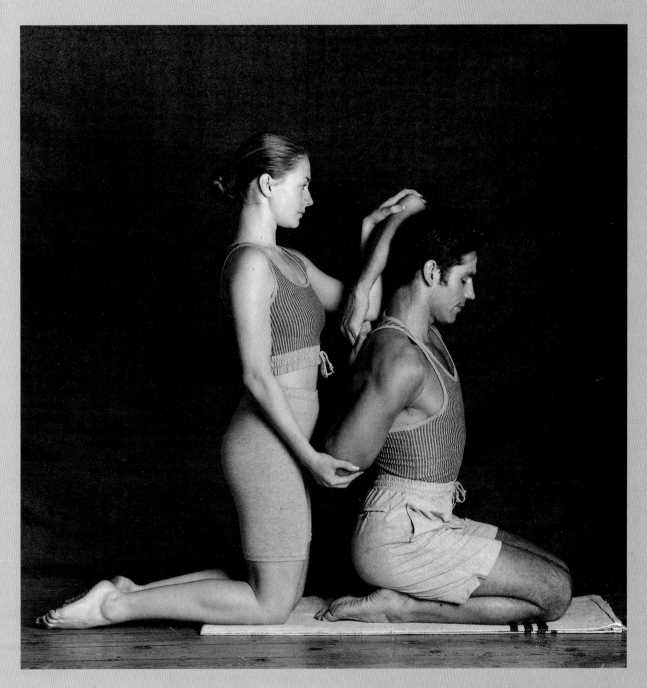

Partnered cowface

The pulled: Kneeling on the floor, raise your left arm above your head, perhaps using your right arm to tug it gently up a little higher, so that the left side of your body is stretched. Bend your left elbow, so your forearm is lowered behind your head, and, holding your left elbow with your right hand, nudge your left arm a little lower, increasing the stretch in your shoulder, but making sure your left elbow points up. Bring your right arm around and up, aiming to clasp hands. If your hands cannot quite reach, hold onto your shirt. Remember to keep your back straight.

The puller: Kneeling upright behind your partner, take hold of the raised elbow with your left hand. Rest your elbow on your partner's back near the shoulder to give yourself leverage. At the same time, take hold of your partner's lower elbow with your right hand. Gently pull your partner's upper elbow back and down while pulling the lower elbow back and up. Hold for 20 seconds, listening carefully to your partner's body. Release the elbows and both relax, then repeat with your partner changing arms. After relaxing again, switch roles.

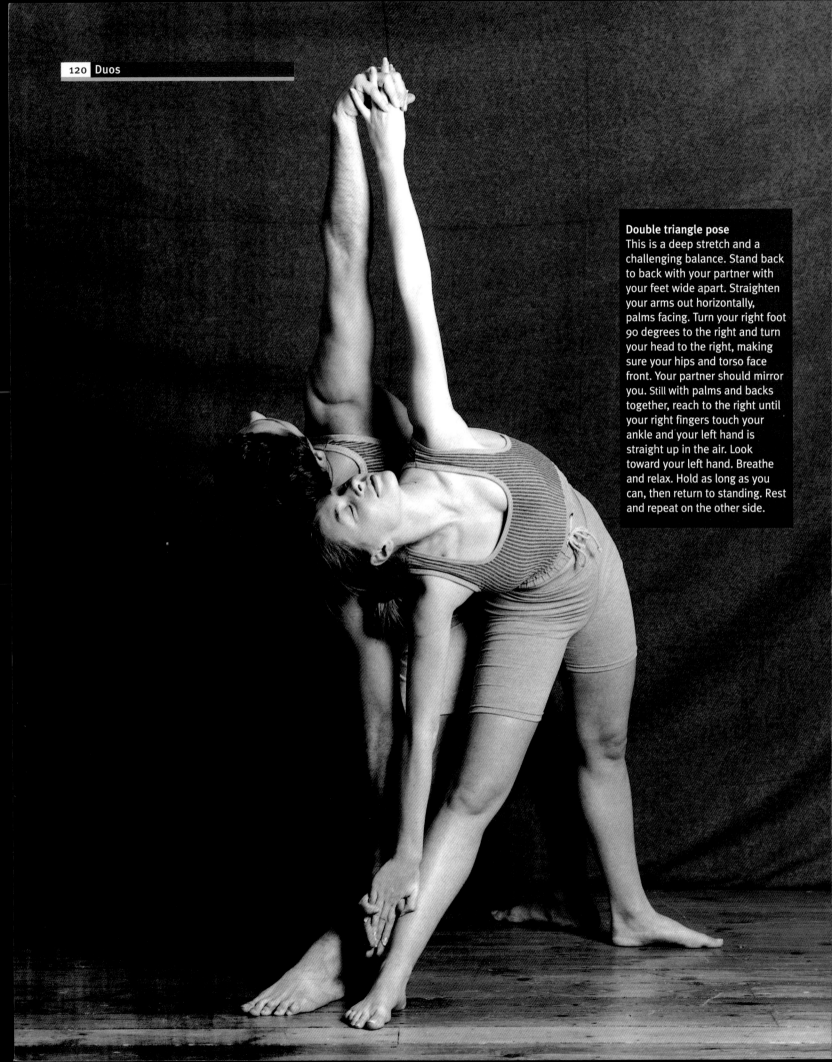

Double triangle pose
This is a deep stretch and a
challenging balance. Stand back
to back with your partner with
your feet wide apart. Straighten
your arms out horizontally,
palms facing. Turn your right foot
90 degrees to the right and turn
your head to the right, making
sure your hips and torso face
front. Your partner should mirror
you. Still with palms and backs
together, reach to the right until
your right fingers touch your
ankle and your left hand is
straight up in the air. Look
toward your left hand. Breathe
and relax. Hold as long as you
can, then return to standing. Rest
and repeat on the other side.

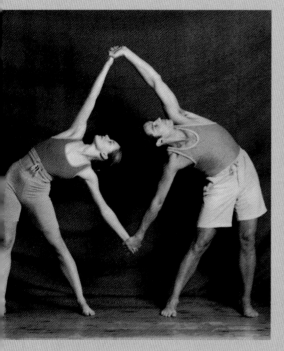 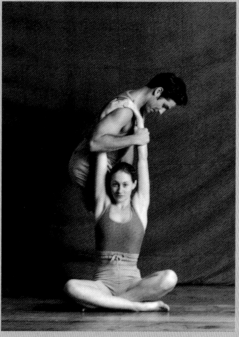 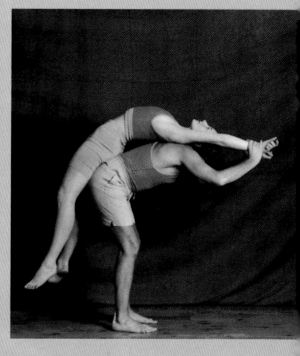

Two person crescent moon

Stand next to your partner, both facing forward.
You should stand about a foot apart, but this
distance will really depend on how easy you
both find the exercise. You will adapt to each
other's needs. Hold your partner's nearest hand
and, standing tall with your feet about hips'
width apart, lift your outside arm and stretch it
over your head until you can hold your
partner's other hand.

Without twisting in the upper body, push your
hips away from your partner, feet flat on the
floor. You should both be making the shape of
the crescent moon. Hold for 30 seconds. To
enhance the stretch, turn your head to look at
your raised hands. Straighten up and unlock
your fingers before repeating on the other side.

Partnered shoulder lift

This is a very dynamic exercise for both
partners. The pulled partner will feel a
satisfying stretch in the arms, shoulders and
back, while the puller will work the side and leg
muscles.

The pulled: Sit cross-legged on the floor and
clasp your hands above your head, elbows
straight but not locked. Relax and enjoy.

The puller: Stand behind your partner at right
angles to your partner's back, with your right
knee bent and resting against your partner's
back. Gently wedge your right shoulder under
your partner's hands and hold their arm.
Carefully shift your weight onto your left leg,
pulling and lifting up and back against your
partner's hands. Hold for 20 seconds, relax,
and repeat on your other side.

Coal lift

This is a fantastic way to stretch and release
your lower back. Ideally this exercise should be
done with a partner who is roughly your size,
but if you are careful, any two people can try it.
Begin by standing back to back and decide who
is going to lift first. Raise your arms in the air.

The lifter: Grab your partner by the wrists.
Bending your knees so that your partner's
buttocks rest in your lower back, gently bend
over until your partner's feet are off the floor. It
is essential that you keep your knees bent at all
times. You can gently rock sideways to enhance
the stretch. When you are finished, lower your
partner gently to the floor before releasing.

The lifted: Let your partner lift you off the
floor, trying to relax completely, concentrating
on your head, neck, and the lower back.
Breathe deeply and trust in your partner.

Rest for a moment before switching roles.

With your baby
duos

Young babies are very demanding of time and attention, and it can be difficult to find quiet, peaceful time to yourself. But even the youngest babies can exercise with you – in their own way. They may simply sleep in your arms as you take advantage of their comforting weight and presence to enhance your stretches. Or you can place them near you and interact with them as you work. Think of lying your baby between your arms as you do the Cat Arching (see page 55) or similar stretches, or holding her in your lap as you try other positions that allow you to remain sitting upright. Remember to hold your baby quite firmly, so that she feels secure, and to support her head carefully. Try to keep your movements smooth and gentle, which will be calming for her. And just as when you work with any other person, you must judge your baby's mood carefully – if she is fretful, you may find that distracting, and it may be better to do something else for a while. By the same token, if you are tense or finding the exercises difficult, your baby will sense that. But if you are both enjoying yourselves, then relax and have fun.

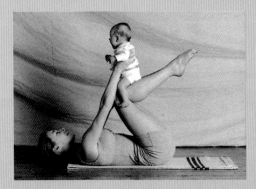 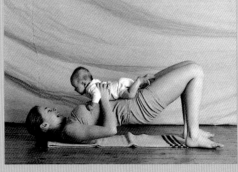 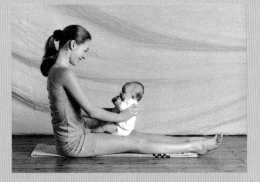

Shin rock
Lie on your back on the floor with your legs in the air, bending your knees so that your shins are parallel to the floor. Keeping your knees together, balance your baby on your shins. As you hold firmly on to your baby, raise your shins from 90 degrees to 45 degrees and back again. Rock your baby up and down in this way 10 times before relaxing.

You may want to improve the exercise by keeping your tummy muscles tight throughout the exercise, but whatever happens, your baby will enjoy the gentle rocking motion.

Baby on the bridge
This is a variation on the basic bridge pose (see page 53) with your baby resting on the bridge formed by your raised body.

Begin lying on your back on the floor with your knees bent and your feet hips' width apart. Rest your baby on your chest and hold her lightly. Lift your pelvis, trying to raise it as high in the air as possible. Hold this position for about 15 seconds, then come down slowly, placing one vertebra on the floor at a time, starting from the top of your spine. Breathe deeply and relax. Repeat five times.

Hip waddle
This is another exercise you can do with or without your baby, but it is much more fun when your baby comes along for the ride.

Sitting comfortably on the floor with your legs stretched straight out in front of you, your ankles together, and your feet flexed, hold your baby upright in your lap. Then, keeping your back straight and your tummy in, propel yourself by slightly raising and shifting forward or backward one buttock at a time. Waddle forward about 10 times, and then waddle backward about 10 times.

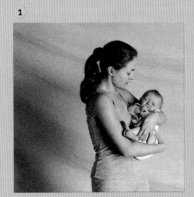 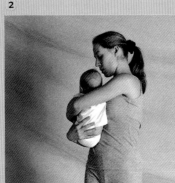

Standing twist
This is a popular stretch that will work your back and amuse your baby. Stand on the floor with your baby in your arms and your feet hips' width apart. Keeping your back straight and hips facing forward at all times, swing your baby to the left until you feel a twist in your back (1). When you can go no further return to your starting position and then repeat on the right-hand side (2). Repeat this sequence 10 times.

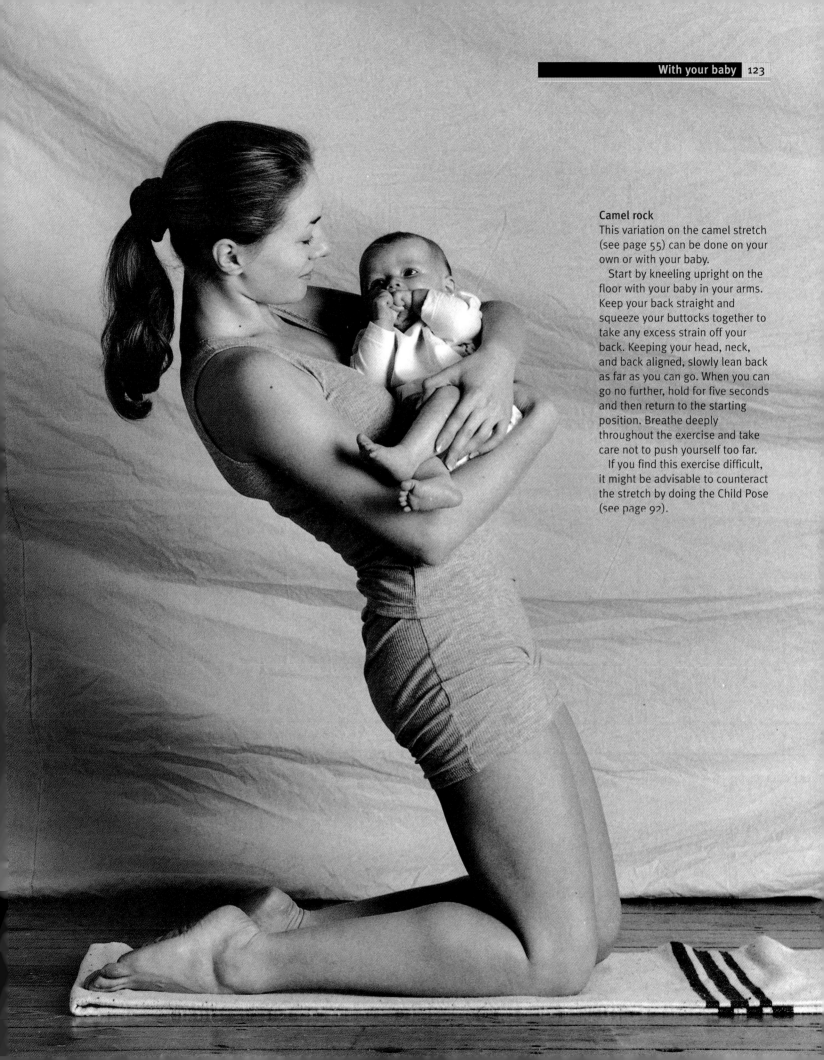

Camel rock

This variation on the camel stretch (see page 55) can be done on your own or with your baby.

Start by kneeling upright on the floor with your baby in your arms. Keep your back straight and squeeze your buttocks together to take any excess strain off your back. Keeping your head, neck, and back aligned, slowly lean back as far as you can go. When you can go no further, hold for five seconds and then return to the starting position. Breathe deeply throughout the exercise and take care not to push yourself too far.

If you find this exercise difficult, it might be advisable to counteract the stretch by doing the Child Pose (see page 92).

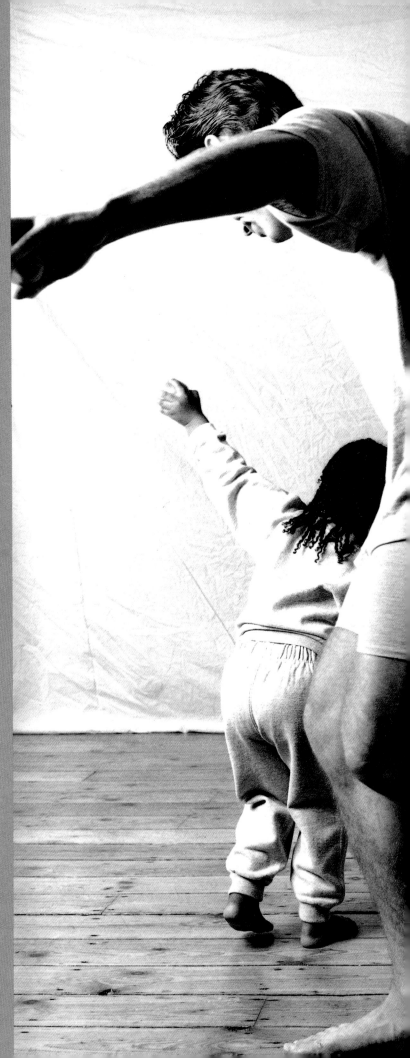

With your child
duos

It has long been recognized that time spent with young children can be very therapeutic – poets have compared it to spending time in bright sunshine. So why not combine the benefits of regular gentle stretching and exercise with spending enjoyable time with your children? If you have put off exercise before because it seemed that your children have not allowed you the time for it, this is the chapter for you. Of course, children may not be aware that they are exercising: babies may sleep in your arms, while older children may delight in the new type of game.

Indeed, many of the exercises described here and elsewhere in the book are things kids do unconsciously as they play. But although children have natural flexibility and posture, the exercises will help to improve their coordination and strength. Meanwhile, you can enjoy the exercises in ways not possible on your own or with your partner. The added fun and laughter with your child will help you to relax and get more out of the stretches.

As you undoubtedly know, children are notoriously fickle, and you will have to be ready to change your stretch at short notice to hold your child's interest. Feel free to improvise with other exercises in the book. Remember: your children are much more flexible than you, so don't stop listening to your own body just because they find it so easy. Above all, keep it fun and playful.

Chicken wings

This is a wonderful shoulder exercise to do with kids, not least because everyone can have fun clucking like a hen as they do it. Standing facing each other, make fists with your hands and place them in your armpits. Then, either standing still or walking around the room, flap your arms vigorously up and down.

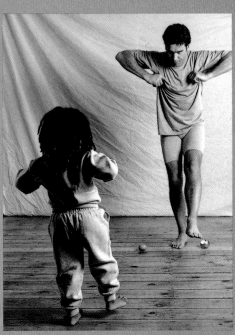

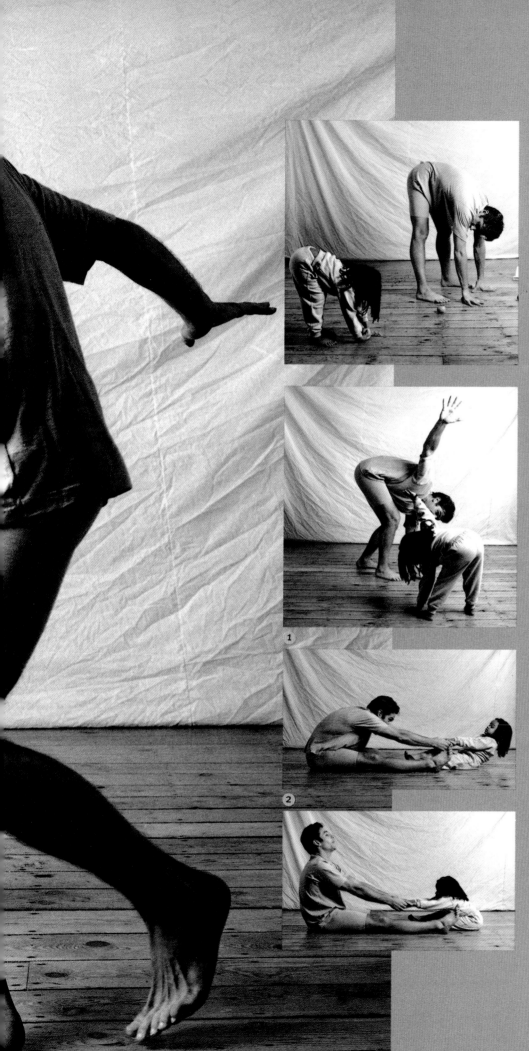

Elephants

Begin standing side by side, with your feet hips' width apart. Tip over from the waist and, without locking your knees, place your palms on the floor. Your child will probably find this easy, but you may have to bend your knees to reach. Relax, with your upper body hanging down from your hips.

Keeping this stance but trying to hold your legs as straight as possible, lift your right hand and foot, and step forward, moving your hand in front at the same time. Do the same with your left hand and foot and repeat so that you walk around the room. You should now look like Mowgli copying the marching elephants in Walt Disney's "The Jungle Book." Continue for as long as is comfortable and fun.

Windmills

This movement combines a gentle standing forward bend with a spinal twist. Bending over freely from your waist, reach down and touch your left foot with your left hand. Raise your right hand in the air and look up at it. Hold this position for as long as you are comfortable, breathing deeply. Repeat on the other side without standing up straight in between. When you are comfortable with this stretch, try to switch arm positions more quickly, without straining your back – or falling over. Do not be surprised, however, if this dissolves into laughter. As an advanced variation, you can touch your left foot with your right hand and vice versa.

See-saw

Sit on the floor with your feet straight out in front of you and your child sitting in the same position opposite you. Letting your child's feet rest inside your ankles, reach forward and take hold of their hands. Now gently pull them toward you so that they bend forward as far as they can, while you lean back as far as you can, without letting go of their hands. Then do the swing the other way round so that you lean forward and your child leans back (1 and 2). You can continue to see-saw backward and forward for as many times as you and your child want, just as long as you both find it comfortable – and it stays fun.

Sports warm-ups

A proper warm-up should prepare your body for the more vigorous movements it will need to perform during a sport, at the same time as it focuses your mind on the activity to come. The stretches specific to your sport will enhance your flexibility and performance, and minimize the risk of injury.

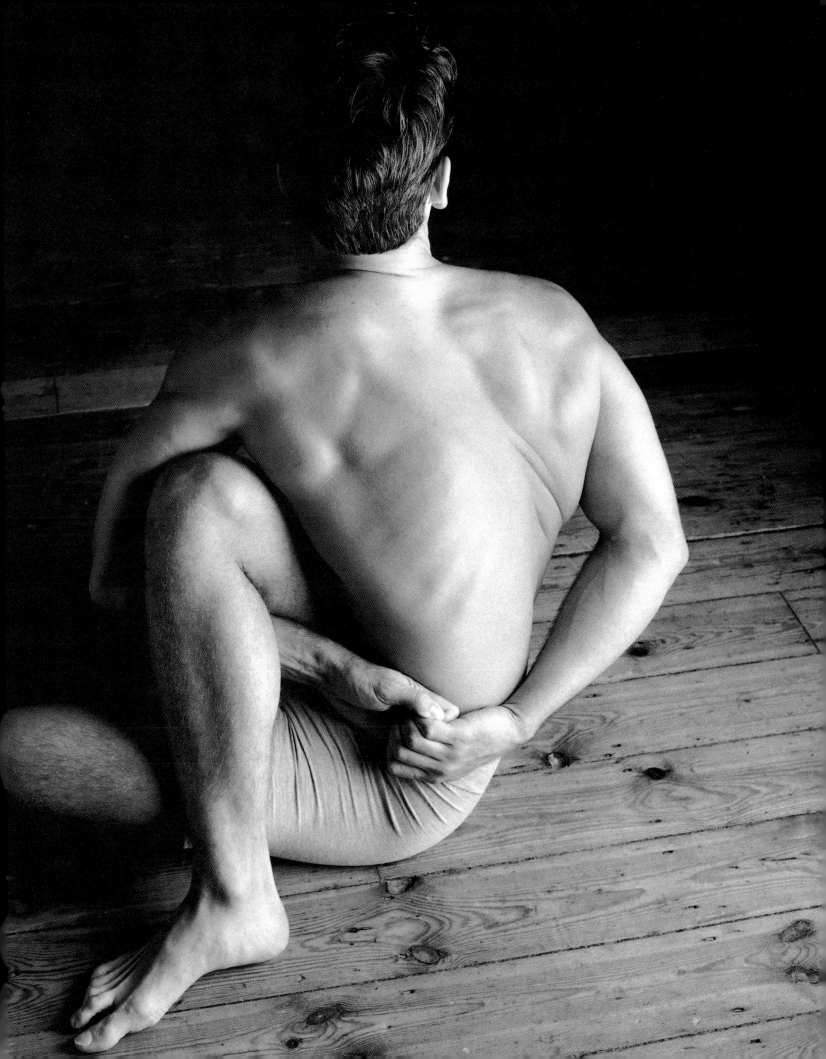

Sports warm-ups
general advice

Although gentle stretching will undoubtedly make you feel and look better, aerobic exercise is also an important part of any fitness plan. Some people choose individual exercise, like swimming or running, while others prefer games, either team sports like basketball or soccer, or racket sports like tennis and squash.

All too often people think that because they are going to exercise when they begin the game or start the run, they do not need the additional work of the warm-up. There seems to be a belief that warm-ups are for professional, not recreational, athletes. In fact, nothing could be further from the truth.

The warm-up prepares your body for the more vigorous movements it will be required to perform during your chosen activity. A warm-up is almost more important for the occasional sportsperson, whose body is less used to strenuous activity, than it is for the professional with a finely-tuned body.

In many people's minds, playing sports is associated with the "no pain, no gain" philosophy – that you have to push yourself beyond your limits to do your best. But this is not true. The body has amazing potential when it is free and flexible, and pain and exercise are not synonymous. This chapter suggests exercises for specific sports that should form the core of your warm-ups. The flexibility they encourage will help you to prevent injury or strain as you perform at your best.

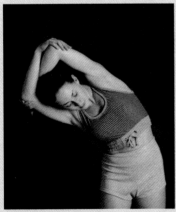
Elbow clasp side bend, page 135

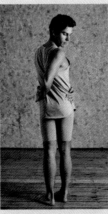
Standing twist, page 136

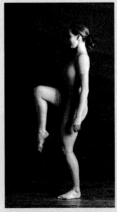
Prancer, page 131

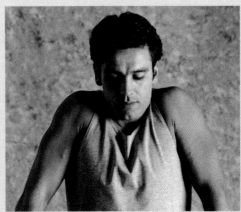
Shoulder shrug, page 137

In the sports warm-up, you work the muscles and joints in a relaxed manner to ease them into the kind of movement you will want them to perform during the game or during the run. The warm-up should also focus your mind on the activity, improve coordination, and generally let you begin your sport without strain.

1 Begin the sports warm-up by literally warming the body up – gently jog, walk, or skip for five minutes.

2 Follow this with some basic stretches such as shoulder rolls, ankle rolls, arm and leg bending, and hip rotations.

3 Now you can go onto the stretches for your chosen sport. The stretches for running (pages 130–31) should be part of a warm-up for any activity involving running.

4 Smoothly incorporate your sport into the warm-up: start with easy hitting in tennis or relaxed passing or heading in soccer, or running at a slow pace.

5 Finally, the cool-down is just as important as the warm-up. After play, always finish up with five minutes of gentle jogging and some simple stretches. Let yourself breathe deeply for as long as your body wants to.

Running
warm-up exercises

Some sporting activities, especially those involving running, are instinctive – they are not something you need to be taught to do. For this reason, it is easy to fall into the trap of not taking the warm-up seriously. But this would be a big mistake.

In running, your legs do most of the work, and many of the warm-up exercises focus on them. However, it is also important to include your feet and ankles. Although they will be protected if you wear well-designed footwear, they remain vulnerable to stresses and strains, especially on the road.

Keep in mind that your whole body participates when you run well. It is all too easy to tense your arms and shoulders, so you must work them gently and keep them consciously relaxed throughout the following exercises. To finish your warm-up, remember to jog up and down in place for a while.

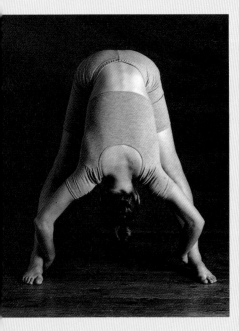

Triangle forward bend
Standing with your feet wide apart, bend forward at the waist and let your arms dangle toward the floor. Then bring your hands through your legs and hold behind your ankles or your calves, depending on how low you can reach. Gently try to pull your head through your legs. Breathe deeply and relax.

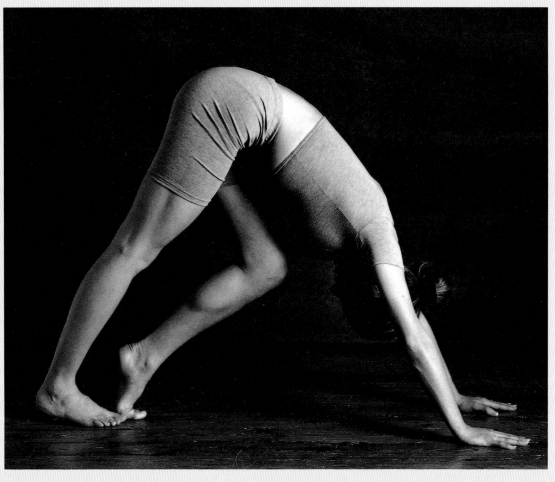

"On your mark"
Bend over from the waist and, keeping your knees loose, place your hands on the floor about three feet in front of you. Bend your left knee, raising yourself onto your left toes, and shifting your weight at your pelvis, then repeat on the other side. You should feel a stretch in your lower back as well as in your legs.
   To make the stretch more dynamic, you can vary this by moving your legs and alternately lifting your feet slightly from the floor, as if you were running in place.

Crouching thigh stretch

Crouching on your toes, place your hands on the floor slightly in front of your knees. Stretch your right leg straight out behind you, resting on the toes of your right foot. Keeping your arms and your right leg straight, think of allowing your hips to sink down toward the floor. This should cause you to feel a stretch running all along the front of your right thigh. As you breathe out, you can feel your hips sinking lower. If you can, hold on to this position for 20 seconds before repeating the exercise with your other leg. Try to work up to holding the stretch for 30 seconds.

Standing hamstring stretch

Raise your right leg, rest your right heel on the seat of a chair, or against a wall, and flex your foot. Place your right hand on the top of your thigh and run it down your leg toward your ankle, keeping your back straight, your head up, and your foot flexed. When you feel a pull in the back of your thigh, hold for 10 seconds, and then change sides. Alternate your legs until you have done 10 on each side.

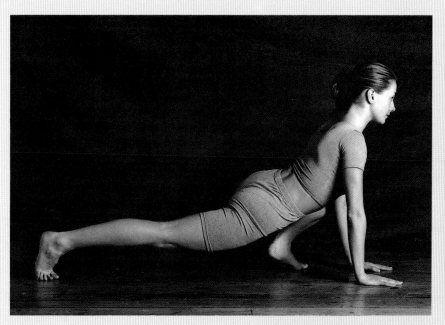

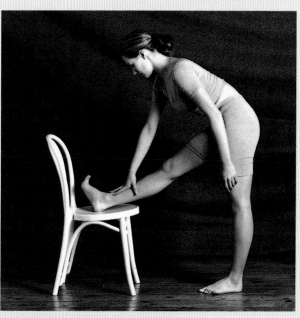

Crescent stretch

Keeping your feet flat on the floor and hips' width apart, raise your left arm and bend it slowly over to the right, without bending forward or backward at the waist. You should feel a strong stretch all along your left side. Hold this position for 10 seconds then switch sides. Do this twice on each side.

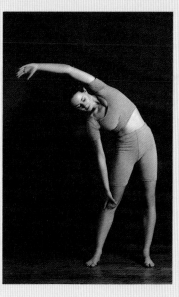

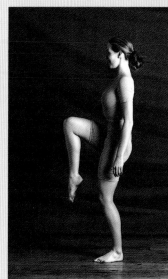

Prancer

Jog in place, raising your knees as high as you can on each step, being careful to keep your arms still by your sides.

Swimming
warm-up exercises

The power of water to relax as well as stimulate muscles makes swimming the perfect sport for people seeking all-round fitness and health. Unlike most sports, it uses all the major muscle groups, toning the body, and breathing and lung capacity can also be greatly enhanced by regular practice.

If you have been unlucky enough to have suffered an injury, a gentle swim can be the best way of working your way back into regular exercise. This does not mean that the warm-up is less important than it is for other sports. You may be less likely to injure yourself in water, but flexibility is still essential. Your arms, shoulders, and thighs work hard in all swimming strokes, and it is best to spend a little time before you swim concentrating on warming up your joints.

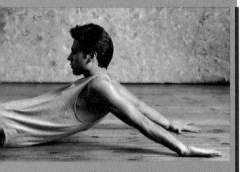

Palm-up shoulder stretch
Sitting on the floor with your feet stretched straight out in front of you, turn your palms up, and place the back of your hands on the floor by your hips with your fingers pointing away behind your back. Slide your palms back and away from you, until you feel a pull in the front of your shoulders. Relax in this position for at least 30 seconds, making sure that you keep your shoulders dropped and your neck relaxed.

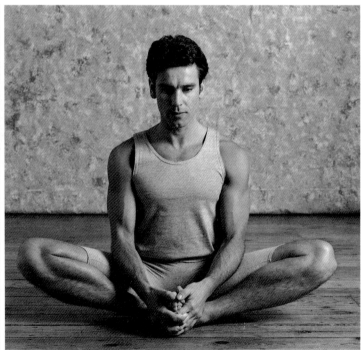

Butterfly
Sitting on the floor with your knees bent, put your feet together so that the soles are touching. Holding your feet with your hands, pull them toward you, trying to get them as close to your groin as you can, without slouching in the lower back. Gently push down on your thighs with your elbows, or lightly bounce your knees up and down to get them as close to the floor as possible. The ultimate aim is for you to get your knees to touch the floor. Remain in this position for between one and three minutes, and then relax.

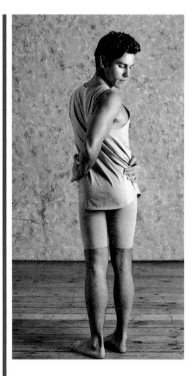

Standing twist
Standing with your feet hips' width apart, thighs and knees facing forward, and shoulders level, twist your pelvis and upper body so you look behind you. Reaching around with your arms, try to twist a little further with every breath. After 30 seconds, reverse the twist.

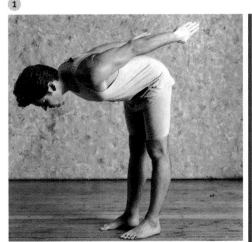

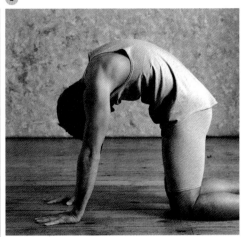

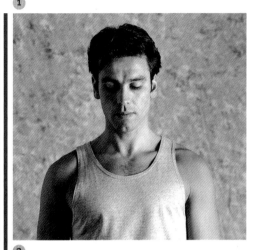

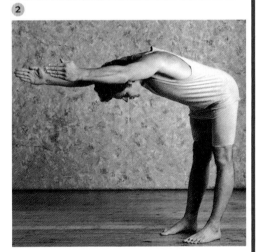

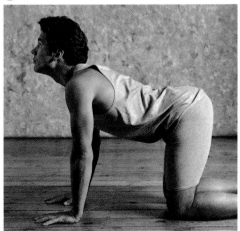

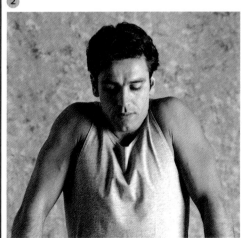

Pendulum

Standing with your feet hips' width apart, bend over from the waist until your upper body is more or less parallel to the floor but you are not straining at all. If the position is not that comfortable, raise your body slightly until it is. Swing your arms freely from your shoulders, aiming to get them higher than your hips on the backward swing (1) and over your head on the forward swing (2). Keep your body still, focusing the movement in your arms and shoulders. Repeat at least 10 times, enjoying the free and easy movement.

Cat arching

Kneeling with your hands on the floor directly under your shoulders, arch your back upward to hunch it and drop your head (1). Then curve your back downward to hollow it, raising your head up (2). Do this about 10 times.

Shoulder shrugs

Standing with your arms relaxed by your sides, lift your shoulders up and squeeze them toward your ears. Hold this position of tension for a moment, then let your shoulders go, allowing them to drop back into their natural position. Relax and breathe out, and as you do so, think of relaxing your shoulders a little more. Don't try to force this relaxation – the simple power of suggestion will be enough to let your shoulders release that little bit more.

Racket sports
warm-up exercises

The element of one-to-one competition in racket sports makes them satisfying to play and great fun. To play well, however, you have to combine good hand-eye coordination with flexibility, strength, and stamina. Your strength and stamina can only develop through specialized training methods. But your flexibility – the ability to stretch high or low to hit the ball – is vital at every skill level. Your warm-up should focus on your arms, hands, and thighs. It is essential to prepare the body for the twisting and turning it will have to do in a game. A thorough warm-up will exercise both sides of the body equally, so that they become equally developed. These warm-up stretches are also useful for sports such as baseball or cricket.

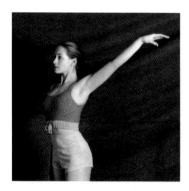

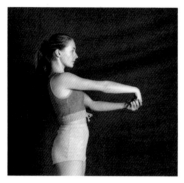

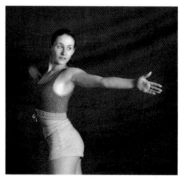

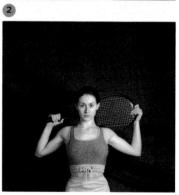

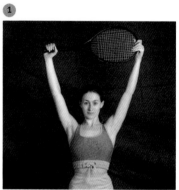

Arm circles
Standing firmly on the floor, rotate your arms in big, slow, controlled circles, moving from the shoulder. Do three circles in one direction before reversing the rotation to do three in the other.

Wrist pull
This simple stretch should help you to avoid tennis elbow. Hold your right arm straight out in front of you at shoulder height, with your palm facing down. With your left hand, hold your right hand and push your right palm toward your body. Hold for as long as is comfortable then switch hands.

Weather vane
Standing with your feet hips' width apart, place your right palm on your upper chest and extend your left arm out horizontally at shoulder height with your palm open and facing forward. Keeping your neck long and your shoulders relaxed, rotate your upper body in a gentle, controlled movement so your left arm swings behind your back as far as it will go without straining. Return to the starting position, change arms, and repeat on the other side. Aim to keep your hips facing forward, concentrating the twist in your back. Repeat the stretch five times on each side.

Racket stretch
Standing with your feet hips' width apart, hold your tennis racket gently at either end in front of you, with palms down. Slowly raise the racket, keeping your elbows straight and arms extended, until you are reaching straight above your head (1). Rest a moment before bringing your arms and the racket down behind your back (2), making sure the racket stays horizontal. Relax, then reverse the movement, returning the racket to the front of your body. Repeat three times.

Backward bend
Separate your feet a little wider than your hips for better balance, and place your hands on your thighs. Tightening your buttocks, stretch gently backward as far as is comfortable, making sure your head goes back to keep your neck in alignment with your spine. You should feel the stretch both in your upper back and in your abdominal muscles.

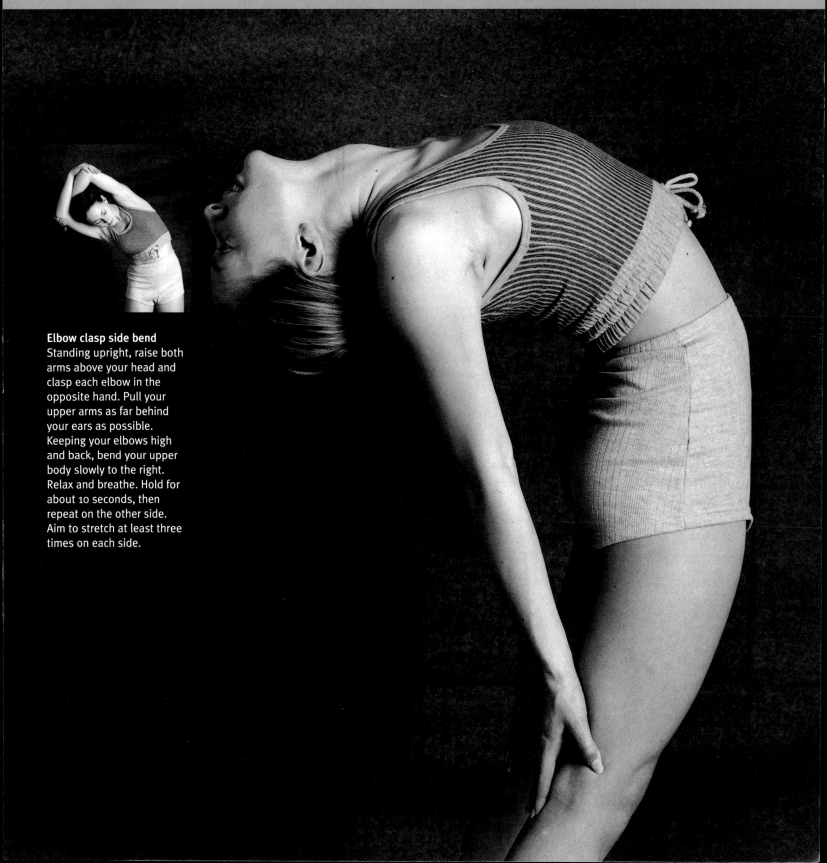

Elbow clasp side bend
Standing upright, raise both arms above your head and clasp each elbow in the opposite hand. Pull your upper arms as far behind your ears as possible. Keeping your elbows high and back, bend your upper body slowly to the right. Relax and breathe. Hold for about 10 seconds, then repeat on the other side. Aim to stretch at least three times on each side.

Ball sports
warm-up exercises

Ball sports like soccer, touch football, basketball, or baseball make a variety of demands on the body, requiring a comprehensive warm-up. They often combine a steady run to stay in the action, with bursts of sprinting. Thus, it is important to add an aerobic element to your warm-up, perhaps varying sprinting with running in place. During a game, it is often after sprinting that you will need great precision for kicking, catching, or throwing, and the flexibility and balance you develop through a warm-up will help you achieve this. Some ball sports involve physical contact. As a result, flexibility in the back, hips, and thighs is very important: hamstring, calf, and thigh stretches are very useful. Stomach exercises are also recommended if you want to play regularly. The stretches suggested here are an ideal place to begin, whichever ball sport you may wish to play.

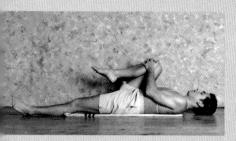

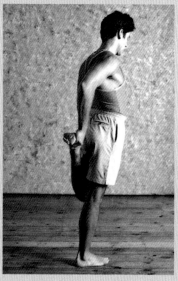

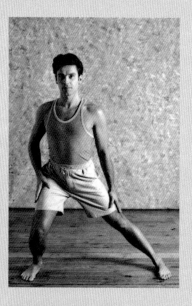

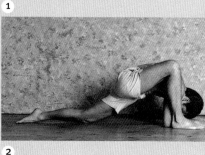

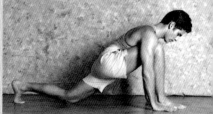

Head to knee stretch
This is a slightly more difficult version of the knee to chest stretch. Begin by lying on the floor and, clasping your right knee with your hand, pull the knee toward your chest. Lift your head and try and touch your knee with your forehead. As an enhancement you might like to try to touch your knee with your nose or ear. After about 30 seconds, relax and repeat on the other side.

Thigh stretch
Stand with your feet hips' width apart. Bend your left knee and, reaching back, hold the inside of your left foot with your right hand. Keep upright and pull your left foot toward your buttocks, taking care to keep your knee pointing to the floor. Hold for 20 seconds and repeat on the other side. Repeat the whole sequence three times. If you have trouble balancing, it may help to rest your free arm against a wall for support, keeping your elbow straight and arm horizontal. Always remember, of course, to stay as upright as possible.

Sideways groin stretch
Standing with your feet two or three feet apart, bend your right knee, feeling the stretch in your left inner thigh. Make sure you keep your body upright. After 15 seconds reverse the stretch.

Lunge
Begin on your hands and knees on the floor. Lift your right foot and place it flat on the floor on the outside of your right hand. Keeping your left foot relaxed and your left knee on the floor, try to place your elbows on the floor adjacent to your foot. Ideally you should be able to place your forearms flat on the floor in front of you (1). Relax in this position for 30 seconds, allowing your hips to sink toward the floor before repeating on the other side. If you find this difficult leave your right arm outside your foot, placing your hand flat on the floor (2).

Sitting spinal twist

Sit on the floor with both legs straight in front of you and your spine upright. Bend your right knee, and put your right foot down on the left side of your left knee. Bend your left knee and bring your foot near your body. Put your right hand on the floor behind your right buttock, with your elbow straight. Lift your left arm and, without bending your elbow, bring it over your upright right knee and place your left hand on your right leg. Turn and look as far as you can over your right shoulder, thinking of raising your lower back. Hold for 30 seconds, release, and switch sides. When you feel strong and supple, reach through your knee with your left hand and clasp hands to intensify the stretch.

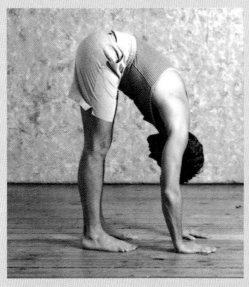

Standing forward bend

Standing with your feet hips' width apart, tip over from the waist and reach down to your feet, but do not lock your knees. You should feel like your upper body is hanging down from your hips. Keep your weight evenly distributed across your feet and, with each breath, relax your stomach muscles and let your back get looser. When you have had enough, slowly roll up, thinking of straightening your back one vertebra at a time.

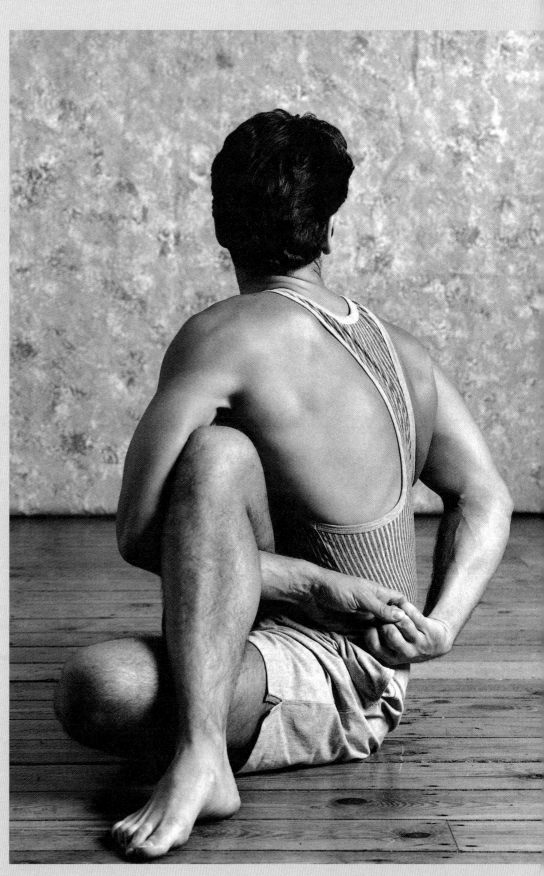

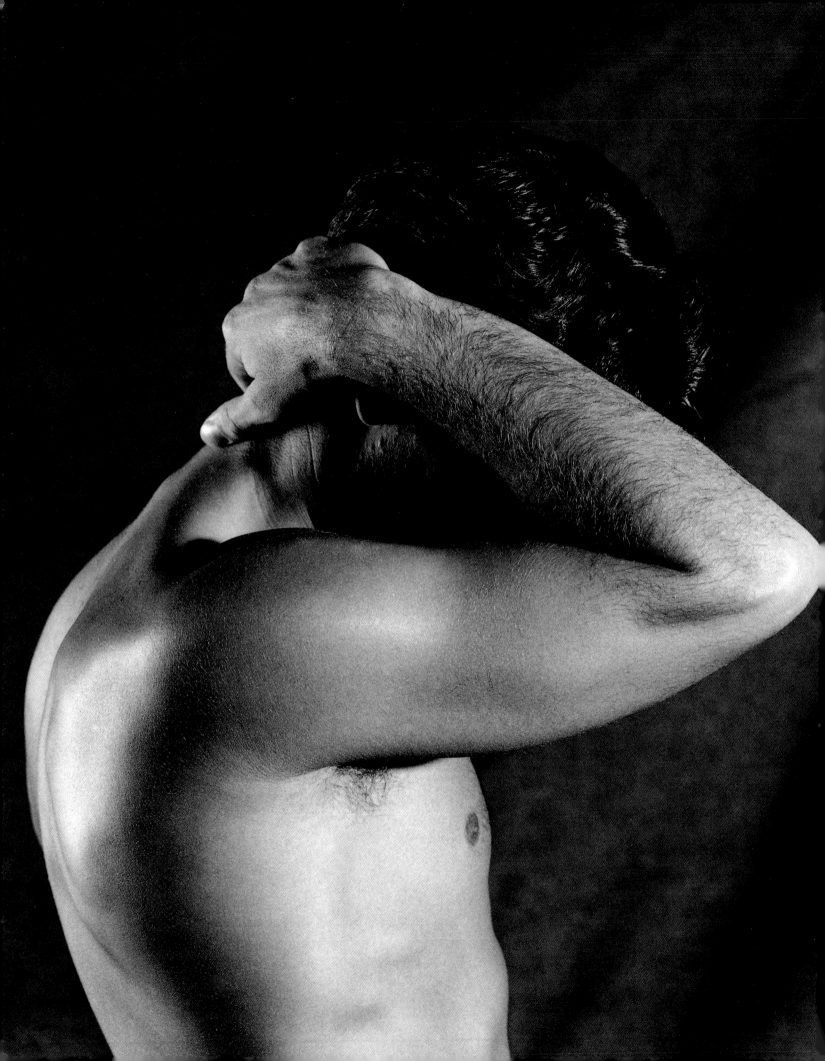

Recommended reading

Barlow, Wilfred *The Alexander Principle: How to Use your Body Without Stress* (Victor Gollancz, London, 1990).

Brown, Mary Eleanor *Therapeutic Recreation and Exercise* (Thorofare, NJ, Slack Inc, 1990).

Chee Soo *The Chinese Art of T'ai Chi Ch'uan* (San Francisco and London, Aquarian Press, 1984).

Clarke, Penny *Taking the Plunge: Swimming for Fitness* (London, Boxtree, 1994).

Evjenth, Olaf, and Jern Hamberg *Autostretching: The Complete Manual of Specific Stretching* (Afta Rehab Förlag, Sweden, 1989).

Feldenkrais, Moshe *Awareness Through Movement* (Arkana, New York and London, 1990).

Fuchs, Viktor *The Art of Singing and Voice Technique: A Handbook for Voice Teachers, for Professionals and Amateur Singers* (Calder and Boyars, London, 1963).

Harrow, Fiona *The Massage Manual* (Headline, London, 1992).

Humphries, Christmas *Concentration and Meditation* (Element, Inc., Massachusetts, 1993).

Iyengar, B K S *Light on Yoga* (Schocken, New York,1977; Thorsons/Aquarian Press, London, 1991).

Lao-tzu (lived *c.*6th century BC) *Cultivating Stillness* (translated and with an introduction by Eva Wong; Shambala Publications Inc., Boston and London, 1992).

Le Shan, Lawrence *How to Meditate* (Little, Brown and Company, Boston, 1988).

McCallion, Michael *The Voice Book* (Faber and Faber, London, 1988).

McNamara, Sheila and Dr Song Xuan Ke *Traditional Chinese Medicine* (Penguin, London and New York, 1995).

Millman, Dan *The Inner Athlete: Realizing Your Fullest Potential* (Stillpoint Publishing, New Hampshire, 1994).

Morrison, Malcolm *Clear speech: Practical Speech Correction and Voice Improvement* (Pitman Publishing Ltd, London, 1977).

Pisk, Litz *The Actor and His Body* (Harrap, London, 1975).

Richer, Paul *Artistic Anatomy* (translated and edited by Robert Beverly Hale, Watson Guptill Publishers, New York, 1971).

Rodenburg, Patsy *The Right to Speak* (Methuen, London, 1992).

Terry, Paul E, and Allan C Kind *It's Your Body: An Up-to-Date Guide to Healthy Living and Preventing Medical Problems* (Chronimed Publishing, Minneapolis, 1992).

Van Lysebeth, André *Yoga Self Taught* (George Allen and Unwin Press, London, 1988).

Waterstone, Richard *The Living Wisdom of India* (Little, Brown and Company, Boston and Macmillan, London, 1995).

Whiteford, Barbara, and Margie Polden *Postnatal Exercises: A Six Month Fitness Programme for Mother and Baby* (Century Hutchinson, London, 1990).

Index

Acknowledgments

The commissioned artwork on page 17 (the human skeleton) and all commissioned photographs © 1995 Duncan Baird Publishers. The photograph on page 9 is reproduced with the kind permission of the British Library, London (Add 26433b).

Sarah Clark MCSP SRP is a chartered physiotherapist. She trained at the Middlesex Hospital, London, and has a special interest in orthopedic and outpatient treatments. She currently works at a private hospital in London.

Liliana Djurovic MCSP SRP is also a chartered physiotherapist. She trained in Belgrade, Yugoslavia, and has a special interest in back and neck pain and sports injuries. She has worked in England for five years and currently works at a private hospital in London.